Praise for *Ossm~~~ ~ ~~~~ ~~~~~* *Household Guide to Appalachian Folk Healing*

"Jake Richards has given the folk magic community a gift by bringing back into circulation Ossman and Steel's collection of important remedies and prayers. Moreover, he has also provided the context for the work through his ongoing commentary. Richards allows the text to speak for itself while also giving explanations and insights from lived experience that fill in the blanks. For the many folks that have had the magic in their families buried or forgotten, this book provides a bridge that would otherwise be difficult to cross. There is both a familiarity in reading the contents, which speak to what many of us grew up hearing in whispers or snippets, as well as information that is likely to be new and aide in growing anyone's repertoire of folk magic. This book is likely to become a touchstone for many folk magicians, healers, and those living in the Appalachian diaspora looking to connect to these traditions."

—Aaron Oberon, author of *Southern Cunning*

"Jake Richards's annotated edition of *Ossman & Steel's Classic Guide* provides the rare opportunity to explore a scarce and culturally significant work on the ritual healing traditions of the Pennsylvania Dutch, who were influential throughout Appalachia. In the reverent voice of a contemporary practitioner, Richards guides readers through this classic healing manual, offering explanations and insights into the inner workings of this folk tradition. *Ossman & Steel's Classic Guide* is also the only known historical work of Pennsylvania Dutch ritual healing written by a mother and son—Ann Ossman and Isaac Steel—underscoring the traditional wisdom in valuing the contributions of both genders in the healing arts."

—Patrick Donmoyer, author of
Powwowing in Pennsylvania

"As a seasoned powwower in the manner of the Pennsylvania German Christian folk tradition, I have always been familiar with the Ossman and Steel work. It is a perfect example of how powwowing was welcomed by our southern neighbors and made workable by the slight alteration of rituals and charms to fit more closely with their southern Appalachian folk Christianity. I highly recommend to all students of folklore studies Jake Richards's updated *Ossman & Steel's Classic Household Guide to Appalachian Folk Healing* with commentary to add context to the rituals and charms. This work is important as it is a true testament of the state of historical folk magic in the Appalachians during the 19th and 20th centuries and has influenced the traditions of conjure and root work in Appalachian folk Christianity for nearly two hundred years."

—Robert Matthew Phoenix, author of
The Powwow Grimoire

OSSMAN & STEEL'S

CLASSIC HOUSEHOLD GUIDE TO

APPALACHIAN FOLK HEALING

ALSO BY JAKE RICHARDS

Backwoods Witchcraft: Conjure & Folk Magic
from Appalachia

Conjure Cards: Fortune-Telling Card Deck and Guidebook

Doctoring the Devil: Notebooks of an
Appalachian Conjure Man

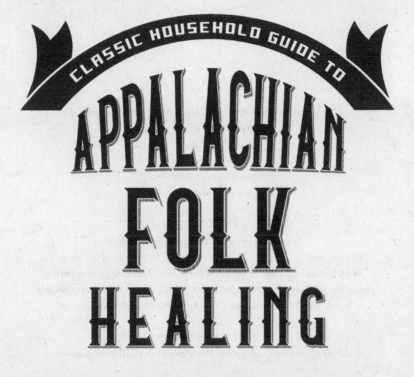

OSSMAN AND STEEL'S

CLASSIC HOUSEHOLD GUIDE TO

APPALACHIAN FOLK HEALING

A Collection of Old-Time Remedies, Charms, and Spells

INTRODUCTION & COMMENTARY BY
JAKE RICHARDS

FOREWORD BY
SILVER RAVENWOLF

WEISER
BOOKS

This edition first published in 2022 by Weiser Books, an imprint of
Red Wheel/Weiser, LLC
With offices at:
65 Parker Street, Suite 7
Newburyport, MA 01950
www.redwheelweiser.com

ISBN: 978-1-57863-753-9
Library of Congress Cataloging-in-Publication Data available upon request.

Cover and text design by Sky Peck Design
Typeset in Arno Pro

Printed in the United States of America
IBI

10 9 8 7 6 5 4 3 2 1

CONTENTS

FOREWORD

The sweat ran.

The sun blazed.

They coughed in the swirls of sand and dirt. The convoy rumbled along a road of tire tracks on earth. Someone made a joke. Laughter. Shouts. A cacophony of ear-splitting sounds. Nostrils contracted and tear-filled eyes widened. Right hand immediately slapped to the chest—subconscious comfort at what lay beneath the uniform. Weapon in hand, she did her duty.

One minute he was walking across the compound toward the mess tent, and the next, he heard the bellow of, "Incoming!" He ran to shelter through billowing dust just as the bomb exploded right where he previously stepped. He let out a "Ha!" of relief, his fist immediately thumping his chest. Subconscious comfort at what lay beneath the uniform. Weapon in hand, he did his duty.

What do these two people have to do with this book? Why do we care that they touched a hand to chest, willing courage to blossom within themselves? What was it that lay beneath the uniform that others could not see?

Let's travel back in time to 1990, when a young woman, a harried mother of four, can't sit still in a wooden chair.

She believes she is about to uncover yet another historical link in the chain of her research: work that weaves together the practice of using intelligent energy, prayer, therapeutic touch, and the power of the word into a unique system of energy healing. Of great interest is how this system of practice has traveled throughout the country and how this folk magick has changed with the influence of each practitioner, community needs, cultural influence, historical events, and eclectic personalities.

What this mother looks for today is a chapbook published in 1894 out of Wiconisco, Pennsylvania, a small township in the rural coal country of Dauphin County. Wiconisco and the surrounding areas were harnessed with low pay and difficult living conditions resulting from the area's primary industry—coal mining. Needs and desires of the common folk birthed this chapbook: the hope of good health, good fortune, happy marriage, and a long life free of anxiety and trouble. Her interest is two-fold: How the practice of Braucherei flowed with the movement of the people, settling where it was most needed, and how it was embraced by mining families as well as farming families.

Her heart thumps. Her breathing quickens. She wears the white gloves the librarian gave her, the palms of her hands moist beneath the cotton. Finally, the librarian returns, smiling. "Yes, we have a full copy. You are in luck! Follow me."

Taking a deep breath and returning the smile, the woman trails after the librarian into a small viewing room that contains a table and two chairs. The book she wanted to view sat in the center of the table. She can't believe her luck.

"Please do not take off the gloves while handling the volume," says the librarian. The young woman takes one look at the book, thrills running up and down her spine. "May I have a copy?" she asks, daring to hope they would allow it. "Of course!" the other woman says. "It will take about an hour or so. Would you like to come back?"

"No, I'll wait," I say.

The book was *Ossman & Steel's Guide to Health or Household Instructor*.

Thirty years later I would send my copy to Jake Richards, who has brought new life to this classic text in this book. And the work continues to flow to the people.

• • •

My name is Jenine Trayer, but most folks call me by my pen name—Silver RavenWolf. My books, including those on folk magick, are published throughout the world. My daily magickal work is called Braucherei (historically known as Pow Wow), a folk healing energy system. I am a descendant of Brauchers and a practicing Braucherin (from the root *brauche* meaning to use, to need, to practice, to employ) in South Central Pennsylvania. I was trained in the art by Preston Zerbe.

Whew! What a mouthful, right?

I am, at this writing, sixty-five years young. For thirty years my work has included efforts in the healing of body and mind, honoring and working with one's ancestors, aligning an individual's spirit to embrace all their talents so they can move forward in a positive way, practices to encourage success, and protection of people, animals, and property. From blessing wedding bouquets for long and happy marriages, to creating blessed baby blankets, to stitching protective and healing dollies and spirit animals, to painting colorful hex signs for the welfare of one's family, I have immersed myself in the spirit-filled process of living a life filled with energy practices. I have assisted in the education of hundreds of such practitioners throughout the years as a result of personal training and group work. I have given talks and seminars on the subject to audiences of all ages, cultures, and religions. I know that anyone with an open mind who believes in positive intent can practice this energy healing system no matter their race, gender, age, cultural background, or religious preference.

The "work" belongs to everyone.

I don't know if any of that makes me an expert, but there you have it.

What has impressed me most about Jake is his sincerity in the practice of folk study and implementation. I have found him to be straightforward and concise in his handling of magickal topics. He is a shining star. One of those people that glitters and gleams to the energy-aware. I was happy to send him my copy of *The Guide to Health* which I procured so long ago. Jake is gifted. Compassionate. His introduction and notes to the reader are beautifully written, carrying valuable information that should not be overlooked. His cautions are valid. His observations on-point.

Does this stuff work?

Jake reminds you that "Such remedies are given here only for historical and educational purposes to retain the wholeness of the work and should in no way be attempted." This does not mean we can't learn the foundational energy work from those who came before us. The chants and charms may remind you of your childhood, bringing back pleasant memories of a simpler time. Some of you will say, "I remember when that old man on the street opposite ours took the thrush from my sister's mouth and blew it away! She never got it after that, but I have no idea what he said while he was doing it!" or "Yep, he blew out the burn." "Yes! She got rid of my warts!" "My brother suffered horribly from colic—neighbor lady took hair, put a tiny hole in the wall and sealed it up! My brother never got it again!" Usually followed by, "Even my mom couldn't hear what the practitioner was saying. I wish I knew."

Oh! I quite forgot! Little old ladies do that sometimes. Why did the soldiers put a hand to their chest? See page 27! Can't stand the suspense? Okay, I'll tell you. Both carried a Himmelsbrief (Letter from Heaven) fashioned by myself and my friends in a small waterproof pouch. These letters were blessed in ritual and dressed with scented oil before being rolled, sealed, and presented to the wearer.

Who were these soldiers? My children—who are alive and well today. And the work carries on.

Peace with the Gods

Peace with Nature

Peace within!

In service,
—SILVER RAVENWOLF
(also known as Jenine Trayer)

INTRODUCTION

The book you now hold in your hands is part of a centuries-old tradition of American frontier living. Faith and healing in America have always gone hand-in-hand, especially among mountaineers and others living far away from cities and towns. The rugged terrain of the Appalachian Mountains warranted that the pioneer ancestors had to figure things out on their own and quickly. Thankfully, when they settled in these mountains they already had the most important qualities in hand: their hope, courage, and self-reliance. That spirit still lives today. Folks then doctored with roots and herbs and prayers— that's how they survived. Whether in the hills of Pennsylvania or deep in the dark hollows of North Carolina, everyone was, and to a varying extent still is, their own doctor.

Whether emigrating from Germany, France, England, Scotland, or Ireland, the people who settled in the Appalachians brought with them their spiritual beliefs. Notable among these were the mystic beliefs brought over by the Pennsylvania Dutch through West Virginia. They held strong ideas regarding the heavenly bodies and the astrological forces they have over the body, as well as a traditional practice of magic and healing.

There were many healing traditions developed in and around Appalachia: on the mid-portion of the mountain range you had *powwow* doctors, essentially faith healers who healed with laying on of hands and spoken biblical charms; Hexes or witches who sent malicious curses on people and livestock; and the Hexenmeister, the witchdoctor who doctored people and animals suffering from witchcraft. The southern end of the range was much the same, though the terms varied: Power doctors, being a southern corruption of the word *powwow*, who healed by prayer in like manner; witches; witchdoctors who removed the witches' work; and the conjurors, those who were for hire in the magical arts and sought to bring about money, success, love, or ruin to enemies. And Appalachia also had its share of fortune-tellers—charlatans, some trustworthy—with methods employed varying between dowsing sticks or rods, playing cards, crystal balls, and the like.

The practice of healing in Appalachia was and is based on the belief in the fundamental interconnectness of all things, from plants and animals, to people and the stars that hang overhead. It's believed that since God has created everything and has deemed it "good" that all natural things (or most) can be used for medicine in one way or another. As God has given to people dominion over the earth, this also includes people's inherent dominion over the diseases that plague them. However, belief in this dominion doesn't stand at the forefront of Appalachian people's relationship with the hills and mountains.

There is a Cherokee story that speaks to this point, a story popular throughout the region. The story retells how people first came to the mountains from the stars. Upon hearing the news the mountains moved and made room, creating valleys for people to live in. The animals and plants agreed to help the humans by supplying hides for clothing, wood for shelter, and bones for tools, since humans were without sharp teeth, thick fur, or other natural tools of survival. This close relationship between people and their natural surroundings has continued on today—something is given for that which is taken. Likewise, this belief in animism endured and influenced the development of Appalachian Christianity. God speaks through nature. Everything in nature is marked with a sign by God of how it might be used to aid us. The notion of divine healing put down deep roots here with many a healer traveling around laying on hands and curing people under the command given in John 14:12, KJV:

Verily, verily, I say unto you, He that believeth on me, the works that I do shall he do also; and greater works than these shall he do; because I go unto my Father.

The names of Christ, God, Mary, the Apostles, and the Angels are called upon to relieve the ailments and trials of man where God's Will gives leeway. As such, the charms that some saw as prayers, and recipes contained herein often call upon the Holy Trinity and draw on narratives of biblical characters that come to aid the sick and poor. Faith is the key here. Faith must be had by both the healer and the patient. With children and animals, those who can't comprehend fully the rites taking place for their betterment, the faith of the parents or the owner of the beast is imperative. Christ himself required faith in order to heal the blind or lame. In Appalachia that faith is still strong today and can be recognized through prayers and prayer cloths, foot washings and anointing still practiced by many churches here.

• • •

Growing up, I remember my grandfather Gene, a Free Will Baptist preacher, displaying with the use of a Bible verse the power to stop bleeding or curing thrush in a child because he never laid eyes on his father. Nana likewise had her charms, such as one that will be found in this book as "A Sure Cure for Headache" (see page 54). Years ago, when I was speaking with her about the things Papaw did, she mentioned he used a "steel book." Me being thirteen years old at the time, I had no clue what she was referring to. To be honest, it called to mind the *metal* steel and I wondered exactly how such a tome might be created. It wasn't until years later that I learned that Nana was likely referring to *Ossman and Steel's Guide to Health*, a book on the Pennsylvania Dutch tradition of *Powwowing* or *Braucherei* (ritual healing traditions), known in Appalachia simply as "trying," from the root *brauche*, meaning to try, use, or treat with medicine.

German-speaking immigrants migrated to Pennsylvania in the 1700s and then down the mountain range, introducing this healing tradition down the Appalachias. But not many things in southern Appalachia families were written down, maybe a scribble here and there in a family Bible or on an index card hidden among an ocean of recipes in a box but that was about it. Mostly, things on healing or other family *work* were taught orally, with the notion they had to be shared in special circumstances, only shared with, for example, a person of the opposite sex, in order for the next generation to be able to utilize the charm. It was thought that if it was shared with someone of the same sex, the person they taught wouldn't be able to use the charm until the teacher had passed away. However, in the northern end of the range, beginning in about the middle of West Virginia and on up, folks wrote things down and had family manuals of witch doctoring (for curing those victimized by acts of malicious magic) and folk healing. These were passed down through the family, as is the case with the "Dahmer Manuscript," described in Gerald C. Milnes' *Signs, Cures, and Witchery: German Appalachian Folklore.*

• • •

Aside from family recipe books kept in northern Appalachia and from the short and rare scribblings found on the southern end, one book governed all and could be found in many homes across the country: *The Long Lost Friend* by John George Hohman, the most famous American grimoire, which is still in use today. While he received much criticism from others, including his own wife, for sharing such highly kept secrets, it seems it found fertile ground in Appalachia. It has never gone out of print since its first publication in 1820, near Reading, PA. Hohman's book became so popular, multiple versions of the book were published by multiple authors, reprinted in full with only a different title. Hohman's work influenced and spread across the entire region of Appalachia, alongside other works he may have borrowed from, such as Albertus Magnus's *Egyptian Secrets* (a text which my grandfather used). The term "borrowed" is used loosely here, as Hohman likely plagiarized other works in creating his own work, which he says he "assembled" from multiple sources, a common practice in that time.

Not long ago, I started looking for that "steel" book Nana had mentioned when I was thirteen. I soon came to realize that it must have slipped out of time and mind. Very few copies still existed, sitting in archives at libraries while others are stored away in museums never to be used again. Nana and I never learned what happened to Papaw's copy as well. Where he got it or where it went remains a mystery.

So, I became pretty sure I'd never get a glimpse of the book beyond the photo of the cover I found online. That is until a very kind and dear friend, Silver RavenWolf, was able to help me acquire a copy via a PDF she made of it. From there I began to compare what I had learned growing up with the recipes contained in the book. Many practices of disease transference and witch doctoring were uncannily similar to those shared in the South through folklore and family practices. It was obvious at that point that the spirits put it on my heart to help this work live on, not only as a healing bridge between people and God, but also between the north and south portions of our shared beloved hills, to continue to be of use in the aid of both man and beast as a household instructor.

The format of the manual is unique and retained here. Every page is adorned with prominent crosses that stand out on the pages. The manual begins with a prayer, or *Himmelsbrief* ("heavenly letter") for protection—the entirety of Psalm 91, which was allegedly carried by George Washington in war. Many of the other charms are adapted or lifted whole cloth from *The Long Lost Friend* and *Egyptian Secrets*. Others are the authors' creations. The charms cover everything from getting thieves to return stolen goods to bringing a bewitched cow's milk back, from healing wounds and stopping the flow of blood to household remedies using plants and greases.

Many of these botanical remedies still retain a magical value to them, such as healing tumors with a found bone or finding aid with the use of dogwood roots dug in the month of June, notably roots that grow toward the rise of the sun. Some of the remedies call for using dangerous substances, such as gunpowder, turpentine, sulphur, and copperas. The reader must keep in mind that these are very old remedies and come from a time when such substances were in common use in the medical field when there was little scientific evidence to back up any medicinal value to such substances. However, many elders even today can remember their mothers giving them tablespoon doses of turpentine for coughs. While they sometimes worked, sometimes they didn't, and sometimes the end result was death. One can well imagine that many people died because of incorrect dosages recommended by self-proclaimed doctors who learned their practice through such books. *Such remedies are given here only for historical and educational purposes to retain the wholeness of the work and should in no way be attempted.*

Commentary has been added where explanation on method or word usage is needed, where adaptation may be had, or where comparisons can be made between Ossman and Steel's charms and those found orally throughout Appalachia, whether in whole or as fragments, whether directly from the Scriptures, or only from them by word of mouth.

• • •

It's thought that Ossman and Steel cashed in on the powwow fascination after Hohman's *Long Lost Friend* set the stage. In their Preface to the book, they even suggest that a good amount of money can be made by one who takes this book door-to-door either selling the book itself or offering services. However, unlike the stance of the authors, pow-wow traditionally held that no money was to change hands between the patient and the Power doctor, because the Power isn't theirs to charge for. Likewise, in the text Ossman and Steel claim the value of some recipes and cures as worth a hundred dollars or more. This is obviously the sort of exaggerated talk that was common during the time, not only of powwow books but also just about every book on magic or medicine in the day. Numerous medical guides began with stories and beliefs that God has provided a botanical cure for every ailment, if people would but search for them. In old advertisements for magic books such as *The Guiding Light to Power and Success* by Mikhail Strabo or *The Ten Lost Books of the Prophets* by Lewis de Claremont, success and power are said to be achieved by following the instructions held within the texts and, if you have a little faith, you may be able to move mountains as Christ said in his teachings.

Such books were advertised by claiming the reader need not walk in darkness or be powerless, calling on the deep-seated poverty that ravaged rural America at the time. They claimed that they contained secret knowledge, detailing stories and tales of the forces at work that made it possible for the book to end up in the readers hands, along with the occasional sob story of the author, likely given to make him more relatable to the reader. Hohman, for example, described himself as nothing but a poor man ravaged by disease before the special cures in his book came to his possession.

Don't let all these old marketing techniques discourage you however; regardless of the format or matter these be presented in, they are tried and true, well done in the spirit of faith. I have seen many of these work with my own eyes and by my own hands. Faith is the key to it. Even Christ needed faith in order to restore sight to the blind or heal the lepers. Each time they asked him to heal them of their maladies, and each time he stated: "Believe ye that I can do this?" to which all replied, "Ye, Lord, we do." And what was his reply to them then, but, "Thy faith has made thee whole." Christ used this particular word usage many times through the Scripture, especially the reply in Matthew chapter 8: "as thou hast believed, so be it done unto thee." Belief is the key here!

A NOTE TO THE READER

The text of the original publication of *Ossman and Steel's Guide to Health* (1894) is reproduced here unaltered, preserving original spellings, grammar, and so forth. You will also see word usage that reflects the racial contexts and beliefs of the time, such as a recipe allegedly originating from "the gypsies," a term now considered a slur by the Romani people to whom it was applied. The word *gypsy* was then often used to incite fascination in the reader, who was often white, as was done in many texts of the day, magical or medical. Claims such as these were held by many of authors of such books, like John George Hohman, who stated some of his recipes came from the "Book of the Gypsies." This may have been a reference to the *Romanus-Büchlein* (The Little Book of the Roma), or to the Egyptian Secrets, from the German *Aegyptiche Geheimnisse,* whose name was based on the false notion that Roma people originally came from Egypt. This ethnical mysticism is due to the cross-cultural belief that "gypsies," "negros," and "Indians" (locally, even the "Melungeons") held special connection to spirits and plants from which much healing could be learned, thus making the content of such works even more desirable to the western world. This belief was largely based on the color of their skin or the implied exotic origin of the person or people (whether Roma, Melungeon, Jewish, etc.) and was the reason behind this racial and ethnic exoticism that is found throughout American folk magic and healing practices. These claims were put forth as the origin of cures, charms, and receipts (old term for recipes) to further add power in them in the mind of the reader, playing on those racial stereotypes of their day, like the stoic, powerful healing "Indian." The power one has or uses is not related to where they come from or how dark their skin is. Do not let this twisted remnant belief of white supremacy influence your work as a healer or your search for one either.

A note on the authors: Ossman and Steel are identified in the book *Powwowing in Pennsylvania* by Patrick J. Donmoyer and were a mother and son duo. That would make this work one of the only powwow books penned in any fashion by a woman. Issac D. Steel of Dauphin County was a tanner and civil war veteran. His mother, Anne Ossman, is shown on census living with him in 1880. Based on census records and the first publication of this book in 1894, they were fifty-nine and seventy-nine years of age. Shortly after its publication, though, Mr. Steel passed away from heart disease. Issac Steel and Anne Ossman, according to Patrick Donmoyer, were the only residents with those surnames living in the village of Wiconisco, a culturally diverse coal town in the northeastern portion of Dauphin County where Greeks, Russians, Slovaks, and Ukranians found work.

Now, I'll leave you to it. Proceed forth with these words from Christ:

Ask, and it shall be given you; seek, and ye shall find; knock, and it shall be opened unto you.

— JAKE RICHARDS

THE GUIDE TO HEALTH

OR

HOUSEHOLD INSTRUCTOR

BY

OSSMAN & STEEL

WICONISCO, PA.

WRITTEN AND VERBAL
SYMPATHETIC MEDICINES

This first part contains verbal and written charms to be spoken and whispered; hidden, carried, worn around the neck, or pressed to the wound to affect healing in either man or beast. The majority of the charms are followed by three large crosses, as was original in Ossman and Steel's manual and indicates, unless noted otherwise, that the charm is to be done three times and always in the name of the Father, Son, and Holy Ghost. "Sympathetic," the concept that describes the hidden connection between all things—from celestial bodies and physical objects to words and symbols—means here that the charms or word-usage illustrates how you wish the situation to go: so for a broken bone, there are narrative charms of Christ healing the broken leg of a horse, a very tough bone to heal, thereby making a human bone heal easier. Notes are added to give explanation on sympathetic word usage and symbolism where possible and where the authors failed to give adequate instruction. Furthermore, a prominent piece of the original work, which we have kept intact, are the three crosses on many of the pages. These are instructive in nature: when you see them, the charm they accompany is to be repeated, said, or done, three times.

—Jake Richards

INTRODUCTION

In introducing our little book, entitled, *Ossman and Steel's Guide to Health*, we believe we have made something known that will be of much value to our readers. Our aim has been to present in as concise a form as is possible such information which will be useful, and to suggest many hints which, if followed according to our directions, will do a great deal of good.

One point we wish particularly to call our reader's attention to, and that is, that the patient's ailments must be known before treating with our remedies. We have carefully arranged and condensed all the matter, so that you may readily find almost any particular information in regard to *Pow Wowing*, &c., in a very short time. We hope and believe this book will prove itself so full of information relating to everyday life, that after being thoroughly read it will be carefully placed in a handy place for reference, and make for itself an indispensable household companion.

One feature of this book we wish especially to impress upon the mind of our readers, and that is, that every word, and every line, and every page, is true. Few books or pamphlets now published are strictly true. There is a thread of truth in them, but so much of romance and fancy are woven around, that the single thread of truth is lost sight of. We give you the facts, not embellished, not enlarged upon, not exaggerated, but the plain, unvarnished truth.

We hardly deem it necessary to give the names and addresses of those who have been cured by our remedies, but should anyone have the least doubt as to the veracity of our statement, we will take pleasure to convince such ones that every word we say is true, upon receipt of stamped envelope for reply. It is not necessary to commit anything to memory (although it is the better plan), as any intelligent person who has sufficient faith in it (as well as the patient), and who believes there is a Heaven and a Hell, can Pow Wow with the greatest success by simply reading from the book, and by following our instructions. Another point we wish to impress upon the mind of our many readers, and that is, that every word we mention in regard to Pow Wowing is taken from the Scripture, and those who have no faith in the Scripture, had better keep their hands off of our book, as they cannot be cured by this method.

You will note we consider some of our secrets worth ONE HUNDRED DOLLARS. We mean just what we say about this matter. ONE HUNDRED DOLLARS is a mere song for some of them, to say nothing of the many other valuable secrets that can be found in our book.

WE WANT AGENTS EVERYWHERE, of either sex, and we don't hesitate to say that any intelligent person who devotes a little time to the study of this book, and who is not afraid to go from house to house and push the business, we make more money in one day than could be made in one week or more at any other employment. All that is necessary is to show the book, from beginning to end, setting forth each subject, &c., and we feel confident that no trouble will be experienced in effecting a sale, as nearly every person will see at a glance that the book is very valuable, and consequently subscribe for one, notwithstanding the fact that it will be necessary to economize elsewhere in order to obtain one.

Write for circulars and terms to agents, enclosing stamps for reply.

—OSSMAN & STEEL.

1894

A SAFEGUARD AGAINST ALL EVIL.

Carried in the Army as a Protection by George Washington

He that dwelleth in the secret place of the Most High shall abide under the shadow of the Almighty. I will say of the Lord, he is my refuge and my fortress: my God; in him will I trust. Surely he shall deliver thee from the snare of the fowler, and from the noisome pestilence. He shall cover three with his feathers, and under his wings shalt thou trust: his truth shall be thy shield and buckler. Thou shalt not be afraid for the terror by night; nor for the arrow that flieth by day; nor for the pestilence that walketh in darkness; nor for the destruction that wasteth at noon-day.

A thousand shall fall at thy side, and ten thousand at thy right hand; but it shall not come nigh thee. Only with thine eyes shalt thou behold and see the reward of the wicked. Because thou hast made the Lord which is my refuge, even the Most High, thy habitation; there shall no evil befall thee, neither shall any plague come nigh thy dwelling, for he shall give his angels charge over thee, to keep thee in all thy ways. They shall bear thee up in their hands, lest thou dash they foot against a stone.

Thou shalt tread upon the lion and adder; the young lion and the dragon shalt thou trample under feet. Because he hath set his love upon me, therefore will I deliver him: I will set him on high, because he hath known my name, He shall call upon me, and I will answer him; I will be with him in trouble. I will deliver him, and honor him. With long life will I satisfy him, and shew him my salvation.

This must be prayed three time each morning while on your knees, and carried about the person. Those who don't believe every word have no faith in the Bible, and to such it will do no good.

COMMENTARY:

Straight from scripture, this charm is mostly the whole portion of Psalm 91, with little change in the wording. Why they included that it may have been carried by George Washington into war is iffy; possibly due to the fact that a founding father of the United States carrying something like this into war may add power to it, fueled by patriotic and religious values of the time.

THE FOLLOWING MORNING PRAYER REPEATED BEFORE ENTERING ON A JOURNEY, WILL PREVENT ALL MANNER OF ILL LUCK.

O Jesus of Nazareth, King of the Jews, yea, King over the whole world, protect (here state full name) during this day and this night—protect me at all times by thy five Holy Bleeding Wounds, that I may not be seized and bound.

The Holy Trinity guard me, that no gun or firearms, ball or lead shall touch my body, and that they shall be as weak as the bloody sweat of Jesus Christ. In the name of God, the Father, the Son and the Holy Ghost. Amen.

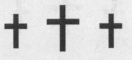

Repeat three times.

COMMENTARY:

This charm would be most appropriate for those embarking on road trips, plane rides, those working among the sick and dying, and so on. The world is full of danger and likewise full of opportunity to preserve oneself. A pound of caution is worth an ounce of cure.

A WELL-TRIED CHARM AGAINST ALL FIRE ARMS.

Three holy drops of blood have passed down the holy cheeks of our dear Lord Jesus Christ, and three holy drops of blood are placed before the touch-hole.[1] As sure as the holy Virgin Mary was pure from all men, so sure shall no fire or smoke pass out of this barrel, or barrels, thou shall not give neither fire, flame nor heat.

---

1   A small hole or vent in early firearms such as muzzleloaders through which the charge was ignited to fire. This word today can simply be replaced with the word *barrel* for the same effect at charming its fire and heat.

I will walk out because the Lord God goeth before me, God the Son us with me, and God the Holy Ghost is above me. In the name of God, the Father, the Son and Holy Ghost. Amen.

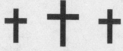

These words must be repeated three times, after which no fire or smoke will pass out of any fire arms. Remember you must see the person or the enemy with fire arms, and stand toward the rise of the sun while repeating the foregoing.

COMMENTARY:

Due to the nature of this prayer, it would be most appropriate in use by soldiers, but may also be used by those who frequently deal in metaphorical wars, especially those within yourself, because in many instances you can be your own worst enemy.

A CHARM TO BE CARRIED ABOUT THE PERSON AS A SAFE GUARD.

Carry the following words about the person, and nothing can harm you in any way: **AWNANIA, AZARIA,** and **MISAEL.** Blessed be the Lord, for he has redeemed us from hell, and he has saved us from death, and he has preserved us even in the midst of the fire.

In the same manner may it please him, our dear Lord Jesus Christ, that there be no fire or danger to me in any way. In the name of God the Father, the Son and Holy Ghost. Amen.

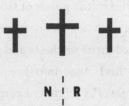

This must be written on white paper, and carried about the person. Care, however, must be taken, so as to mention the person's name who carries it, and also to have it written correctly. This is a sentence not to be played with, and no fun should be made with it, as it is all taken out of the Scripture, and those who don't have faith in the Scripture has better keep their hands off, as it will do no good to that class of people.

A TRUE BENEDICTION AGAINST FIRE OR CONFLICT.

Welcome thou fiery flame, do not extend farther than thou already hast, this I count unto thee as a repentant act. In the name of God, the Father, the Son and Holy Ghost. I command unto thee by the power of God, who created and worketh everything, that thou do cease and not extend any farther, as certainly as Christ was standing on Jordan's stormy bank being baptized by John the holy man; this I count unto thee as a repentant act. In the name of the Holy Trinity, I command unto thee by the power of God, now to abate thy flames, as certainly as Mary retained her virginity before all ladies who retained theirs so chaste and pure; therefore, fire cease they wrath, this I count unto thee as a repentant act. In the name of the most Holy Trinity I command unto thee to abate thy heat, by the precious blood of Jesus Christ which he shed for us and our sins and transgressions; this I count unto thee as a repentant act. In the name of God, the Father, the Son and Holy Ghost.

Jesus of Nazareth, King of the Jews, help us from this dangerous fire, and guard this land and its bounds from all epidemic diseases and pestilence. Amen.

Remarks on the Foregoing.

Those who have this sentence in their house will be free from all danger of fire, as well as lightning. If a pregnant woman carries this letter about her person, neither enchantment nor evil spirits can injure her or her child; furthermore, if any person has this letter in the house, or carries it about the person, they will be safe from the injury of pestilence.

Anyone who has sufficient faith in this sentence, can check the largest fire by simply walking around it three times, each time repeating these words, and making a ring around it on the ground three times also. We don't pretend to say that the fire can be entirely extinguished by this method, but we do pretend to say that the fire won't and cannot possibly get over the rings made on the ground. We invite anyone to build a fire on some wooden floor, at the same time following our directions (the outskirts of the ring made on the wooden floor may be well soaked with kerosene if desired), and be convinced that every word we say is true.

COMMENTARY:

Although its name alludes to a use against metaphorical "heat" in the form of conflict, which they convey as being conflict between persons, it is rather odd that O&S listed so many uses for this one charm but still lacked one for the conflicts it is so partially named for. To further add to this work, I would suggest that you may also keep the letter in your home or at your workspace to keep conflicts between people at bay. If a conflict does occur and you are able to, try to reach a resolution with the letter on the floor and your left foot resting upon it. Even better if both parties participate and place their left foot upon it while facing each other and speaking.

A TRUE BENEDICTION FOR AND AGAINST ALL ENEMIES.

The cross of Christ be with me, the cross of Christ overcome all waters and every fire, the cross of Christ overcome all weapons, the cross of Christ is a perfect sign and blessing to every soul. May Christ be with me and my body during all my life, at day and night. Now I pray to the God the Father for the soul's sake, and I pray to God the Holy Ghost for the Father and the Son's sake, that the holy corpse of God may bless me against all evil things, words and works.

The cross of Christ open unto me; furthermore, blessed cross of Christ be with me, above me, before me, behind me, beneath me, and everywhere before all my enemies visible and invisible. These all flee from me as soon as they know or hear Enoch and Elias, the two prophets who were never imprisoned nor bound or beaten, and who never came out of their power, thus no one of my enemies can injure me, or attack my body, or take my life, in the name of God, the Father, the Son and Holy Ghost. Amen.

✝ ✝ ✝

Repeat three times each morning.

COMMENTARY:

To extend the reach of this charm beyond simple vocalization, you may also be inclined to use it like a glory note or *himmelsbrief* ("heavenly letter") by writing it down on paper and carrying it on the person or displaying it in the home.

A GYPSY SENTENCE TO BE CARRIED ABOUT THE PERSON AS A PROTECTION UNDER ALL CIRCUMSTANCES.

Like unto the Prophet Jonas as a type of Christ, who was guarded three days and three nights in the belly of a whale, this shall the Almighty God as a Father guard and protect me from all evil. **J J J.** This is Jesus of Nazareth, King of the Jews. In the name of God, the Father, the Son and the Holy Ghost. Amen.

✝ ✝ ✝

HOW TO WALK AND STEP SECURELY
IN ALL PLACES.

Jesus walketh with (here state name) he is my head, and I am his limb, therefore, walketh Jesus with (here state name). In the name of God, the Father, the Son and Holy Ghost. Amen.

✝ ✝ ✝

COMMENTARY:

This uses for such a charm as this are numerous and full of possibility, which is the greatest thing about folk magic. You don't fit it, it fits to you. As such, you may pray this three times every day upon waking, have it written and soaked in water to bathe sore legs and feet, or place it beneath the doorstep or porch for a strong foundation in the home.

A SURE REMEDY TO COMPEL THIEVES TO
RETURN STOLEN GOODS.

Early in the morning before sunrise, go to a pear tree, and take with you three screws out of a coffin, or three horse shoe nails that have never been used, and holding them toward the rise of the sun, say: O thief, I bind thee by the first nail, which I drive into thy skull and brains, to return the goods thou hast stolen in their former place.

Thou shall feel sick, and as anxious to see me and the place from which you have stolen, as the Disciple Judas felt after betraying Jesus Christ.

I bind thee by the second nail, which I drive into your lungs and liver, to return the stolen goods to their former place.

Thou shall feel as sick and as anxious to see me and the place from which you have stolen, as did Pilate in the fires of hell.

The third nail I shall drive into thy feet, O thief, in order that thou shalt return the stolen goods to the very same place from which thou has stolen.

I bind thee and compel thee, by the three holy nails which were driven through the hands and feet of our dear Lord Jesus Christ, to return the stolen goods to the very same place from which thou hast stolen them.

In the name of God, the Father, the Son and Holy Ghost. Amen.

✝ ✝ ✝

The nails, however, must be greased with grease of an executed criminal, or other sinful poison. Dragon's blood will answer the purpose, which can be obtained in the drug stores. Care must be taken so as not to drive the nails or screws in the tree too far, or you will kill the thief.

Also, that the nails are taken out of the tree again, or both tree and thief will die. While repeating these words, never drive the nails or screws in the tree until you come to the place where it tells you to do so.

Bear in mind this method must be used before sunrise in the morning, and within twenty-four hours after the goods have been stolen. If tried any other time it will be in vain.

Well worth one hundred dollars.

COMMENTARY:

Also lifted from Hohman's *The Long Lost Friend*, Ossman and Steel's (O&S) variation seems to only change the original prayer a bit, with the word "men" being replaced with "me" in the conjuring of each nail. In the original, this is likely to incite fear and guilt when the thief is around anyone, as if they can see written on his skin that he stole, as opposed to O&S variation which only conjures that in the presence of the conjuror. O&S also includes the substitute of Dragon's blood for the grease of a criminal. The pear tree specified is a special portion of Appalachian charms. Usually when removing something like disease, it is specified to find and utilize a tree which bears no fruit, the reason being the disease will go into the tree and may pass it on to someone else who may eat of the fruit. But here, the fruitful pear tree is called up because the conjuror needs the thief to bear "fruit," or the stolen goods, to him.

ANOTHER METHOD OF BINDING THIEVES.

Thieves, I conjure you to be obedient, like Jesus Christ obeyed his heavenly Father unto the cross, and to stand still. In the name of the Trinity, I command you by the power of God, to stand as still as Jesus Christ stood on Jordan's stormy bank to be baptized by John, and furthermore, I conjure your horse and rider to stand still, and not move any more than Jesus Christ, when he was about to be nailed to the cross.

To release the Father of the church from the bonds of hell, ye thieves I bind you with the same bonds which Jesus Christ our Lord has bound hell, and this ye shall be bound. In the name of God, the Father, the Son and Holy Ghost. Amen.

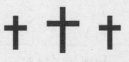

Repeat the foregoing three times. Remember the same words that binds a thief, or thieves, must release them.

THE FOLLOWING IS TO RELEASE STILL BOUND THIEVES.

You horseman or footman whom I have conjured at this time may pass on, in the name of Jesus Christ through the word of God and the will of Christ ride or walk ye onward and pass. In the name of God, the Father, the Son and Holy Ghost. Amen.

✝ ✝ ✝

Repeat these words three times also. Should you try this method of binding thieves, we would advise you to release them within twenty-four hours, unless you desire to kill them.

COMMENTARY:

The portion of killing the thief is interesting here. Although it's not noted, it may be assumed that such charms of drawing thieves out is done in like-manner to other charms in the northern tradition: with the timing of the moon. Thus to draw or pull, it may be done in the growth or wax of the moon cycle. If such is the case, it may be that the longer the thief is compelled, the harder the pull is on his spirit. Taking into account the fact the spirit, or at least a portion of it, may run out of the body due to dire circumstances or trauma, the still-binding of a thief may grow in such power with the moon so as to pull and pull until something is pulled from him, in this case, his life.

HOW TO FASTEN OR SPELL BIND THIEVES.

Say, Christ's cross and Christ's crown. Jesus Christ colored blood be thou every hour good. God the Father is before me, God the Son is beside me, God the Holy Ghost is behind me; whatever is stronger than these three persons may come by day or night to steal me or my property. In the name of God, the Father, the Son and Holy Ghost. Amen.

✝ ✝ ✝

Repeat these words, together with the Lord's Prayer, three times, while walking three times around the property you desire to protect from thieves, and we assure you should the thief or thieves get in the ring, they will not be able to get out until you release them.

Release thieves by repeating the same words as in the other method.

HOW TO PREVENT WITCHES FROM BEWITCHING PERSONS OR CATTLE.

Trotter head, I forbid thee my house and premises; I forbid thee my horse and cow stable; I forbid thee my bed and bedstead, that thou mayest not breathe upon me or anything that belongs to me or my family.

Breathe unto some other house until thou hast counted every fence and post, until thou hast ascended every hill and mountain, and until thou hast crossed every water in the world; and thy dear days may come again into my house.

In the name of God, the Father, the Son and Holy Ghost. Amen.

✝ ✝ ✝

These words must be written on a piece of white paper, and placed in the stable when the cattle are tormented; or placed on the bedstead if people are tormented. This will protect and free all people and animals from witchcraft. Bear in mind that nothing dare be loaned or stolen from house, premises or person until nine days after this has been resorted to, or it will be in vain.

COMMENTARY:

This is a common theme in folk magic across the world: the ordering of spirits or illnesses with impossible tasks that must be completed before they will be able to re-enter or revisit the host of their malice and trickery. This is especially apparent in old folktales regarding the Devil, in which he is told to count every leaf, number every star as it is born and dies, and to braid a rope out of sand. As the task is impossible, the spirit or illness will never return to the host from which it was banished.

ANOTHER GOOD REMEDY AGAINST EVIL SPIRITS.

If any one is troubled with bad people take either a hog or beef bladder before sunrise in the morning, and before conversing with any person; stand with your face toward sunrise and urinate in either of these bladders, then tie it shut as tight as you possibly can, after which fasten the bladder with the urine in the chimney so that it cannot be taken out conveniently.

All this must be done before conversing with any person, and we feel confident that the person who tormented you will never do it again. Care, however, must be taken that nothing is loaned or stolen from the house, premises or person within nine days, or this remedy will be in vain. Do this in the name of God, the Father, the Son and Holy Ghost. Amen.

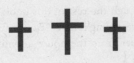

A STILL BETTER REMEDY AGAINST EVIL SPIRITS AND ALL WITCHCRAFT.

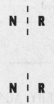

All this be guarded here in time, and there in eternity. Amen.

The foregoing must be written on a piece of white paper and carried about the person. The characters or letter signify: God bless me here in time, and there in eternity. It is supposed that this be sewed in a small new muslin bag, and hung around the neck. Be careful so that nothing is loaned or stolen from the house, premises or person within nine days.

COMMENTARY:

We see this phrasing a lot with these charms, and will continue to through the rest of this book, but I wanted to make a note regarding it here. "Be careful that nothing is loaned or stolen from the house, premises, or person for nine days." Here we see that a guard or protection is put up for a timeframe of nine days, at which point it is presumed that the given charm will have had adequate time to grow in strength to protect the person, much like a crab waiting for his shell to re-harden. During this period, especially if the charm is being done to counteract any witchcraft, it was believed that the witch would come to borrow or take something—which I explain in-depth in my book, *Doctoring the Devil*—so they could regain and retain power over the victim and his household.

HOW TO RELEASE PERSONS WHO ARE BEWITCHED.

Three false tongues have bound (here state Christian name of patient). Three holy tongues have spoken for (here state Christian name of patient). The first is God the Father, the second is God the Son, and the third is God the Holy Ghost. They will give (here again state Christian name of patient) flesh and blood, peace and comfort. Flesh and blood will grow upon your bones again which was lost on you, as surely as the flesh and blood grew on our dear Lord Jesus Christ, so surely will the flesh and blood grow on your bones again.

If any man trampled on you with his horse, God will bless you. If any woman has trampled on you, God and the body of Mary the mother of our dear Lord Jesus Christ, will bless you. If any servant has given you trouble you will be blessed through God and the laws of heaven. If any servant, man or woman, has led you astray, God and the heavenly constellation shall bless. (Here state Christian name of patient.)

Heaven is above thee, earth is beneath, and thou art between. God will bless you against all trampling by horses. Our dear Lord Jesus Christ walked about in his bitter affliction and died. The Jews spoke unto the Son of God as if he had the itch. Then spake Jesus, I have no itch, and none shall have it, whoever will assist me to carry the cross, him or her will I free. In the name of God, the Father, the Son and Holy Ghost. Amen.

✝ ✝ ✝

This must be written on white paper and carried about the person in a small muslin bag. The muslin must never have been wet, or dare a knot be in the thread with which the small bag is made.

HOW TO RELEASE SICK COWS THAT ARE BEWITCHED.

J. The cross of Jesus Christ poured out milk. **J.** The cross of Jesus Christ poured out water. **J.** The cross of Jesus Christ has poured them out.

Write these lines on three pieces of white paper, then take about a half pint of the sick cow's milk, and the three pieces of white paper, together with a small quantity of bone scraped from the skull of a criminal; close it well and put it over a hot fire, and the witch will have to die.

If you take the three pieces of white paper in your mouth, and go out before your house, at the same time speaking three times (any words are preferable), and then give them to your cattle, you will not only see the witch, but your cattle will get well again also.

THE FOLLOWING TO BE GIVEN TO CATTLE IN THEIR FEED AGAINST WITCHCRAFT

SATOR
AREPO
TENET
OPERA
ROTAS

This must be written on white paper, and the cattle made to swallow it in their feed.

HOW TO PREVENT WICKED OR MALICIOUS PERSONS FROM DOING YOU AN INJURY.

DWLLIX IXWX yea, yea, you can't come over. Pontious, Pontious, above Pilate.

In the name of God, the Father, the Son and Holy Ghost. Amen.

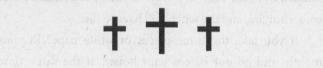

A SURE CURE FOR THE WASTING AWAY OF FLESH ON PEOPLE.

Repeat the following:

Flesh shall grow on (here state Christian name of patient) bones, which is lost and wasted away; as sure as our dear Lord Jesus Christ was born of the Virgin May and laid into the manger, so surely shall the flesh grow on (here again state Christian name of patient) bones again. In the name of God, the Father, the Son and Holy Ghost. Amen.

† † †

Repeat these words three times, each time rubbing over the bare skin of the patient with your hands from head to foot. Remember a cure cannot be affected by this method, unless it is done in either the increase or decrease of the moon.

COMMENTARY:

The comment regarding the moon was not written as well as it could've been. Here, O&S seem to imply that a cure can be effected as the moon wanes and waxes, but not during its fixed points: whether a full moon or a new moon, much like the climax and pivot of a rollercoaster.

A SURE CURE FOR THE DECAY OR WASTING AWAY OF FLESH ON CHILDREN AND GROWN PERSONS.

Do the following on the first three Fridays of the decrease of the moon, and also on the first three Fridays of the increase of the moon. Go over the patient with your bare hands from head to foot, and at the same time look towards the moon, and repeat the following:

What I look at shall decrease, and what I rub over shall increase, as surely as the moon decreases, so surely shall the flesh and blood grow on (here state Christian name of patient) bones again.

As surely as our dear Lord Jesus Christ was born and laid into the manger and moved out of the manger, and arrived at manhood, so surely shall the flesh and blood grow on (here again state Christian name[2] of patient) bones again, and you shall have strength and power again also.

In the name of God, the Father, the Son and Holy Ghost. Amen.

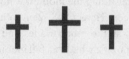

Go over patient with your bare hands from head to foot three times, each time repeating the foregoing.

When pow-wowing in the increase of the moon, say what I look at shall increase, instead of saying what I look at shall decrease.

---

2   "Christian name" throughout the text refers to a person's full name, first, middle, and last.

A SURE CURE FOR STILLING THE BLOOD, NO MATTER HOW FAR THE PATIENT IS FROM YOU, PROVIDING THE CHRISTIAN NAME IS KNOWN.

Repeat the following three times:

Jesus Christ's dearest blood, that stoppeth the blood, in this help (here state Christian name of patient). In the name of God, the Father, the Son and Holy Ghost. Amen.

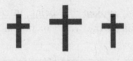

ANOTHER METHOD OF STILLING THE BLOOD ON PEOPLE OR ANIMALS.

As soon as the cut or wound is inflicted, repeat the following:

Blessed wound, blessed hour, blessed be the day on which Jesus Christ was born. In the name of God, the Father, the Son and Holy Ghost. Amen.

✝ ✝ ✝

Remember the forgoing must be repeated three times, and also the Christian name of the patient mentioned. We would advise any one to lay their hand near cut or wound while repeating these words.

COMMENTARY:

Many old charms call upon this special day for various reasons, especially those dealing with healing. Power is held in the reference to this day as it is the day that Creation met Creator, like a second "giving of life" to the universe, but in a more intimate way than the biblical genesis wherein creation is simply spoken into being, in contrast to other gods who produced the world or humans directly from themselves.

A SURE CURE FOR PAINS, OR STILLING BLOOD ON PERSONS OR ANIMALS.

Three holy men went over before (here state Christian name of patient) and they saw (patient) lying in blood and pain, and they spoke and said: Thou shalt live; thou shalt live; thou shalt live. In the name of God, the Father, the Son and Holy Ghost. Amen.

† † †

Repeat these words three times, and at the same time go over patient from head to foot with your bare hands. Then blow your breath over patient three times also.

A SURE CURE FOR STILLING BLOOD WHEN AN ARTERY IS CUT, OR WHEN ALL OTHER REMEDIES OUTSIDE OF OURS HAVE FAILED.

Write the following on a piece of white paper, and lay it over the bleeding wound, and we assure our readers that the blood will cease flowing in a very short time.

I. MI. K. I. B. IP. A. X. V. SS. SS. VAS. I. P. O. UNAY LIT DOM MPER VOBISM.

Do this in the name of God, the Father, the Son and Holy Ghost. Amen.

✝ ✝ ✝

Whenever a woman is about to give birth to a child, let her write these words on paper and have them about the person. It will certainly be of avail.

We invite those who are inclined to doubt our word, to write these words on the blade of a knife, and stab some animal, and be convinced that it is true when we say no blood will flow from the animal.

It give us great pleasure to state that this remedy has saved a many one from the grave, and especially women. We have cured cases that the best physicians even failed to help a particle, after exhausting every effort. We invariably find the medicine of God above all others.

A NEVER-FAILING CURE FOR WILD FIRE, OR ERYSIPELAS, NO MATTER HOW FAR GONE.

Repeat the following:

The wild fire and the outrageous flew over a wagon; the wild fire abandoned, and the dragon sheddeth. Brand go over the sand three times.

In the name of God, the Father, the Son and Holy Ghost. Amen.

✝ ✝ ✝

Repeat these words three times, each time going over naked *patient with your bare hands* from head to foot. Be careful that no one is behind you and the patient, for fear of throwing this terrible disease on others. Powwow for patient three times a day, thus making nine applications.

We have cured the worst kind of cases in a few days' time, and are still doing so from time to time. We are glad to say we have entirely cured cases that have been under the best physicians treatment, and whose remedies only aggravated the disease instead of giving relief.

A SURE CURE FOR SCURVY, DIPHTHERIA, AND SORE THROAT.

Speak the following and it will certainly help you.

Job went through the land, holding his staff close in his hand; God the Lord met him and said: Job, what art thou grieved at? Job said, O God, why should I not be sad, for my throat and mouth are rottening away. Then said the Lord unto Job, in yonder valley there is a well of water which will surely cure (here state Christian name of patient) throat and mouth.

In the name of God, the Father, the Son and Holy Ghost. Amen.

✝ ✝ ✝

The foregoing must be repeated three times in the morning, and three times in the evening. Where it reads, it will surely cure (patient's name). Your breath must be blown in the patient's mouth three times. Hundreds of the worst kind of cases have been cured by this method. A single failure is unknown to us.

A SURE REMEDY FOR HEALING A SORE MOUTH.

If you have the scurvy, or quinsy, breathe your breath in the patient's mouth three times and say: I breathe my breath three times in (here state Christian name of patient). Do this in the name of God, the Father, the Son and Holy Ghost. Amen.

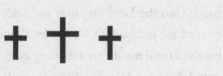

COMMENTARY:

Due to the illnesses this charm addresses, I believe it would be wise to repeat this charm three times a day for three days: once at waking, high noon, and before retiring to bed after the sun has set. Scurvy, or quinsy, is the swelling and bleeding of gums, which is caused by a vitamin C deficiency.

A VERY GOOD REMEDY FOR TAKING FIRE OUT OF BURNS OR SCALDS.

Repeat the following:

Our dear Sarah journeyed through the land, having a fiery hot, hot brand in her hand. The firebrand heats and the firebrand sweats. Firebrand stop your heat. Firebrand stop your sweat.

In the name of God, the Father, the Son and Holy Ghost. Amen.

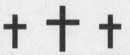

Bear in mind these words must be repeated three times.

HOW TO TAKE PAINS OUT OF FRESH WOUNDS.

Repeat the following:

Our dear Lord Jesus Christ has a great many wounds, and yet He never had them dressed; they did not grow old, or were they ever cut or found running. A man was blind and spoke to the heavenly child as sure as five holy wounds were inflicted on our dear Lord Jesus Christ. In the name of God, the Father, Son and Holy Ghost. Amen.

✝ ✝ ✝

Repeat these words three times, each time mentioning patient's Christian name.

If this remedy does not cure (or any other of our pow-wowing remedies), these is no use of resorting to others, as any one who has faith in the Holy Bible will agree with us when we say that our dear Savior's medicine is above all others.

A SURE REMEDY FOR REMOVING BRUISES AND PAIN.

Speak the following words:

Bruises thou shalt not beat,

Bruises thou shalt not sweat,

Bruises thou shalt not run,

No more than the the Virgin Mary shall bring forth another son.

In the name of God, the Father, the Son and Holy Ghost. Amen.

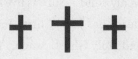

Repeat three times and go over wound with your bare hand from wound to fingers, or from wound to toes.

COMMENTARY:

Here we can see an example of what I call passing rites and transference rites; moving the hands down the body begin-ning from the wound or infliction and moving away from the heart towards the extremities, the hands and feet. This is to essentially "draw" or "pull" the power of the wound out of the body. Usually when rites like this are conducted, especially if the wound is contagious or infected, the healer, once finished, will go immediately to a cold stream of water (preferably one running west) and wash his hands in it to wash away the "residue" of whatever he has pulled or drawn from the patient.

A SURE CURE FOR RHEUMATISM.

Rheumatism come out of the marrow into the bones, out of the bones into the flesh and blood, out of the flesh and blood into the skin, out of the skin upon the skin, from the skin into (here state Christian name of patient's) hair, out of the hair into the green forest, out of the green forest into the dry forest, as sure as our dear Lord Jesus Christ moved out of the manger.

In the name of God, the Father, the Son and Holy Ghost. Amen.

✝ ✝ ✝

The foregoing must be repeated three times, each time going over the patient with your bare hands from head to foot. Then blow your breath over patient from head to foot three times also. We would advise our readers not to pow-wow for any one, unless they have a stronger constitution than the patient.

HOW TO CURE THE BITE OF A SNAKE, NO MATTER HOW FAR THE PATIENT OR ANIMAL IS GONE.

Repeat the following three times, each time going over patient with your bare hands from wound to boot:

God has created all things and they were good. Thou only serpent art damned. Cursed be thou and thy sting.

In the name of God, the Father, the Son and Holy Ghost. Amen.

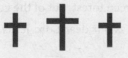

Zing, Zing, Zing.

If the snake has not been killed it will go to the place where the person or animal was bitten and die as soon as this remedy has been used on the patient.

We consider this secret worth the cost of the entire book alone, as it has and will save many a one from the grave. Too much thanks can't be given us for suggesting a remedy like this.

A SURE CURE FOR HYSTERICS, OR MOTHER FITS.

Go over bare skin of patient with your thumbs from the shoulder blade to the pit of the heart, thence across the ribs to the back-bone three times, each time repeating the following:

Matrix Patrix lay thyself right and safe, or thou or I shall on the third day fill the grave.

In the name of God, the Father, the Son and Holy Ghost. Amen.

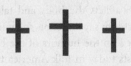

Bear in mind these words must be repeated three times each hour, for three hours, thus making nine applications.

A SURE CURE FOR HEADACHE

Tame thou flesh and blood like Jesus Christ in Paradise who will assist thee, this I tell (here state Christian name of patient), for your repentance sake. In the name of God, the Father the Son and Holy Ghost. Amen.

✝ ✝ ✝

Repeat these words three times, and your headache will soon disappear. Should the headache not cease within ten minutes repeat the words three times again. This, however, is often not necessary.

COMMENTARY:

A variation of this charm was used by my family, and in my experience, has worked the majority of the time with great success. In my family, this charm's aid is multi-purpose and is not limited to only headaches, but may be used for any condition which afflicts the body and takes it out of its natural state, that is to say infection, inflammation, and the like. This is based on the humors of the body. A medical belief still persists today in folk America that the body is composed of humors such as blood, phlegm, and black and yellow bile, which must stay in balance, or the result is illness of some sort determined by whatever humor is out of balance.

HOW TO CURE THE COLD OR INFLAMMATION IN PERSONS.

Speak the following:

Inflammation lose thy color, like Judas lost his color when he betrayed our Lord Jesus Christ.

In the name of God, the Father, the Son and Holy Ghost. Amen.

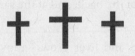

The foregoing must be repeated three times, each time rubbing over the bare skin of the patient with your hands. Then blow your breath over patient three times also.

COMMENTARY:

This charm works best, in my experience, if there is a bowl of ice cold water placed beneath the patient's bed and changed out each time the ice has completely melted, for as long as the charm is repeated until the patient has been cured.

A WELL-TRIED REMEDY FOR HEART BOUND AND LIVER GROWN.

Take warm lard and grease the patient from the shoulders to the pit of the heart, also along both sides of the ribs to the spine of the back.

After this is done, run your thumbs from the shoulders of the patient to the spoon of the breast, thence along the ribs to the spine of the back, and at the same time repeat the following:

Heart bound and liver grown, move from lungs and liver, like our Lord Jesus Christ moved out at the manger. This I do in goodness, so that this will flee from (here state Christian name of patient).

In the name of God, the Father, the Son and Holy Ghost. Amen.

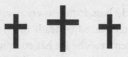

Repeat the foregoing three times. Treat patient on the back likewise, running thumb half way down the back. Remember patient's feet must be toward the rise of the sun, and that the hands and feet must be greased with lard also. This remedy has never been known to fail.

A VERY GOOD CURE FOR THE WEAL IN THE EYE.

Take a dirty plate, if you have none, you can easily dirty one, and the person for whom you have sympathy shall in a few minutes find the pain much relieved. You must hold the dirty side of the plate which is used for eating toward the eye and say:

Dirty plate, I press the weal in the eye
(here state name of patient).

In the name of God, the Father, the Son and Holy Ghost.
Amen.

Repeat these words three times. This remedy has been never known to fail.

A SURE CURE FOR PALPITATION OF THE HEART.

Repeat the following three times: Palpitation be out of (here state Christian name of patient) heart, since our Lord Jesus Christ speaketh with his lips. In the name of God the Father, the Son and Holy Ghost. Amen.

✝ ✝ ✝

The same remedy may also be used for hide-bound. Instead of saying palpitation be out of patient's heart, say hide-bound be off of patient's ribs.

COMMENTARY:

Hide-bound, along with the term "liver grown," identified illnesses where the liver was believed to grow to the body cavity, attaching itself to the "hide" and causing pain and cramping in the upper abdomen. Today this is identified mostly with things like colic. Heartburn, along with hernia and heart failure, on the other hand (due to their like symptoms) were believed to be the result of the heart doing the same as the liver and attaching itself to the body cavity, making it feel rough and congested, which they termed "heart-bound." The same can also occur in animals, especially livestock, for which many a call were made to the local healer.

A VERY GOOD REMEDY FOR CURING SWEENY IN PERSONS OR ANIMALS.

Repeat the following:

Sweeny come out of the marrow in the bones, out of the bones into the flesh and blood, out of the flesh and blood into the skin, out of the skin upon the skin, from the skin into the hair, out of (here state Christian name of patient) hair as sure as our dear Lord Jesus Christ moved out of the manger.

In the name of God, the Father, the Son and Holy Ghost. Amen.

✝ ✝ ✝

Repeat these words three times, each time going over patient with your bare hands from head to foot. This can only be done on the first Friday of the decrease of the moon.

COMMENTARY:

The foregoing charm illustrates how literal folk magic can be while still remaining non-static. Here, the disease sweeny (defined as the wasting away of muscles, especially those in the shoulder) is directed step by step into leaving the patient, without the disease knowing. Much like leaving bread crumbs for a bird, the bird is distracted by each coming crumb and not the direction in which they're heading or being lead. Not even the fact they are being lead to begin with. This way the disease is eased out of the body with little to no struggle from the disease, while also ensuring the session isn't as hard on the patient's body as some other charms may be where the disease is directly moved out.

Other variations continue the directions given to the illness even after the step from the body in total, whether it be to the rocks, from the rocks to the trees, from the trees to the soil, from the soil to the water, and so on, even sometimes directing it to an environment far, far away from the present location such as a desert or tundra.

A FIRST-CLASS REMEDY FOR COLIC, OR WIND COLIC, IN PERSONS OR ANIMALS.

Repeat the following three times, each time going over patient with your bare hands from head to foot:

I warn ye, ye colic finders, that there is one standing in judgement who speaketh just to the unjust, therefore beware ye, ye colic finders.

In the name of God, the Father, the Son and Holy Ghost. Amen.

† † †

This remedy has been tried hundreds of times and never known to fail.

COMMENTARY:

This charm identifies and addresses the different forms of colic or colic-like symptoms under the title Colic Finders, likely a corruption of the German *Feinde* meaning enemies or malevolent entities that carry or bring disease.

HOW TO CURE SWELLING OF CATTLE.

Desh break no flesh. While saying this run your hands along the back of the animal from the head. Do this in the name of God, the Father, the Son and Holy Ghost. Amen.

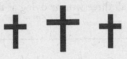

Repeat these words three times.

A BENEDICTION AGAINST WORMS.

Peter and Jesus went out upon the field, they ploughed up three furrows and ploughed up three worms. The one was white, the second was red, and the third was black. Say dead. Now all the worms are dead.

In the name of God, the Father, the Son and Holy Ghost. Amen.

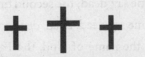

Repeat these words three times.

COMMENTARY:

Much like with the previous colic charm, we see the different forms of worms symbolized in the charm by different colors: white, black, and red, which are very prominent in American folk magic and in folk healing, relate to the different colors of wounds and blood, whether infection, a bruise, or a cut: the colors also correspond to the humors. Here the charm identifies and names each with a color, and concludes with all three worms dying at the command of the one doctoring.

A SURE CURE FOR WORMS IN PERSONS OR HORSES.

Repeat the following:

Three holy men went over the land holding three worms in their hands. The first was white, the second was red, and the third was black. Dead.

Repeat these words three times, each time you say dead hit the patient or animal on the belly with the palm of your hand.

The first time say, dead; the second time say, dead, dead; and the third time say dead, dead, dead are all the worms.

Do this in the name of God, the Father, the Son and Holy Ghost. Amen.

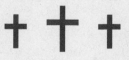

Here we see the same occurring as with the previous charm against worms, with the added action of hitting the patient or beast on the belly, not hard enough to hurt, but hard enough to hurt or kill the worm, as if the worm was outside of the body and physically vulnerable to your touch. Through this action, the worms are killed by the charm.

A SURE CURE FOR FRESH STRAINS ON PERSON OR ANIMALS.

Repeat the following:

Our dear Lord Jesus Christ hung at the cross, and his hanging did not do him any harm, therefore (here state Christian name of patient) strain shall do thee no harm than it did out dear Lord Jesus Christ when he hung at the cross.

In the name of God, the Father, the Son and Holy Ghost. Amen.

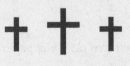

Repeat these words three times, each time going over patient with your bare hands from wound to feet.

COMMENTARY:

One of my personal favorite type of charms is this one, where the human body, being man in the image of God, is likewise related to being in the same condition as that of Christ: barely affected by physical pain as we see in the first verse "his hanging did not do him any harm." While some may call this sacrilegious, being that Christ did feel pain in his sacrifice, I do not see that being the intention here, but rather that he overcame it, even breaking the gates of death and hell, and therefore stands above physical pain. We can see this further in the many road signs that litter the south saying "He lives." With this charm, it may be used for any pain should you substitute the word strain for pain, swelling, and the like.

AGAINST EVERY EVIL INFLUENCE.

Our dear Lord Jesus Christ, thy wounds so red, will guard against death. In the name of God, the Father, the Son and Holy Ghost. Amen.

✝ ✝ ✝

This is to be written on white paper and carried about the person.

HOW TO TREAT A SICK COW AFTER THE MILK IS TAKEN FROM HER, OR WHEN SHE GIVES BLOODY MILK.

Give the cow three spoonsfull of her last milk, and say to the spirits in her blood, ninety has done it and I have swallowed him or her. In the name of God, the Father, the Son and Holy Ghost. Amen.

✝ ✝ ✝

After following our directions, repeat such a prayer as may be deemed necessary.

A REMEDY TO BE USED WHEN ONE IS SICK AND WASTING AWAY IN FLESH WHICH HAS EFFECTED MANY A CURE WHERE DOCTORS COULD NOT HELP.

Let the patient without having conversed with anyone, urinate in a new bottle before sunrise in the morning. Then put nine new needles and nine new pins in the bottle, and close as tight as you possibly can and immediately lock the bottle with its contents in a tight box or chest, after which the keyhole must be well closed with bread or putty.

The key, however, must be carried with the person who locked the box or chest shut. Some one will come to loan, but be careful so as not to loan anything from the house, premises or person within nine days, or this remedy will be in vain. Care must also be taken that nothing is stolen from either of these places.

ANOTHER REMEDY TO BE USED WHEN ONE IS FALLING AWAY IN FLESH, WHICH HAS CURED HUNDREDS.

Let the patient, in perfect soberness and without having conversed with anyone urinate in a vessel before sun rise in the morning. Boil an egg in the urine, and after this is done bore three holes in the egg with a pointy instrument, then carry the egg to an ant hill (commonly called *piss myers*), and the patient will feel relieved as soon as the egg is devoured.

A PROTECTION AGAINST CROSS DOGS.

Repeat the following:

Dog hold thy nose to the ground, God has made me and hound.

In the name of God, the Father, the Son and Holy Ghost. Amen.

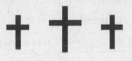

Repeat the words three times in the direction of the dog, then make three crosses on the ground toward him also. Bear in mind all this must be done before the dog sees you. This is to prevent cross dogs from barking or doing any one harm.

OSSMAN AND STEEL'S METHOD OF CURING THE BITE OF A MAD DOG.

First burn the bite with lunar caustic or nitrate of silver, then take one ounce of red chicken weed gathered in the month of June or July, and dried in the shade, put it into a quart of strong brewer's beer, boil it down to one pint and strain through a clear cloth, then stir into the tea one ounce of teriac, so that it will be well mixed. The dose for a man of a strong constitution to be half a pint in the morning and the other half pint the next morning. The patient should fast three hours after taking the medicine. Eat nothing but bread and butter, or bread and molasses for a week or ten days, abstaining from all kinds of meat. Drink nothing but tea. The patient should not get angry nor overheat himself by work. For children and persons of a weak constitution, divide the same quantity into three doses. For animals the quantity must be doubled, and fed in wheat bran warm. This remedy must be used within twenty-four hours after the bite.

HOW TO CURE THE FALLING FITS.

Take a piece of the rope with which a criminal was executed, and sew it in the patient's clothing unknown to him. At the same time take a small quantity of the rope, and make it into as fine a powder as possible, then take an equal part of pulverized licorice, and make into three ordinary pills, coat the pills with refined white sugar or chocolate if desired, and give the patient a pill every three hours. This we assure our readers will permanently cure this terrible disease, provided the patient is not afflicted with some other disease in connection with the falling fits. Be careful so as not to let patient dissolve

pills on the tongue, or let him know what the pills are composed of, or there will be no hope of ever getting cured with
this valuable remedy.

THE FOLLOWING TO BE CARRIED ABOUT THE PERSON AS A PROTECTION WHILE OUT HUNTING.

UT. NEMO : IN. SENSE. TENTAT. DESCE. UDERE. NEMO.

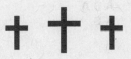

AT. PRECEDENTI. SPECTATUR. MANTICATERGO.

Those who carry this while out hunting need not regret
having got hold of it, as it not only prevents one from doing
your gun an injury so that nothing can be killed, but also
against all manner of ill-luck.

A WELL-TRIED REMEDY FOR CONVULSIVE FEVER.

Write the following letters on a piece of white paper, sew it in a piece of linen or muslin, and hang it around the neck until the convulsive fever leaves:

ABAXACAT
ABAXACA
ABAXAC
ABAXA
ABAX
ABA
AB

If this remedy does not effect a cure there is no use of trying others. It is mostly intended for children, and we would not advise any one to use it where there is but little hope of the patient's recovery, unless you either desire to effect a permanent cure or kill.

A SURE CURE FOR CONSUMPTION, NO MATTER HOW SEVERE, PROVIDED THE PATIENT'S LUNGS ARE NOT TOO FAR GONE.

Take three tablespoonfuls of dog's lard each day, and also eat freely of dog's flesh until relief is obtained. Care, however, must be taken so that the flesh and lard is obtained from healthy dogs. If any one doubts what we say about this matter, and will write us, sending stamp for reply, we will be pleased to refer such ones to parties who have been saved from the grave by following these directions.

A WELL-TRIED REMEDY FOR CATARRH IN THE HANDS, &C.

Take three white onions and roast them in ashes after which peel the outside skin from them. Then take three white lily onions, together with one handful of fresh wild indigo root (commonly called fly bush; it grows in the woods), and after bruising these articles well, put them in a frying pan, together with the three roasted onions, one pint of sweet milk and three tablespoonfuls of wheat flour, and boil it down to a poultice. After this is done make plasters and apply to the diseased parts as warm as the patient can bear it;

always bearing in mind that a new plaster must be added as soon as the other gets cold. Continue on with this until the pain relieves and the affected part becomes white. Should the poultice get hard and stiff, add a little fresh milk occasionally, and keep warming it up in this manner.

To prepare this remedy is a little troublesome, but we guarantee it will cure after all others fail. Cases have been cured by this remedy after doctors fail to give relief, and where it would have been necessary to amputate the hand, had it not been for this valuable remedy.

HOW TO CURE TYPHOID FEVER WHEN ALL OTHER REMEDIES FAIL.

Dig up the roots of white dog wood and wild cherry that are in the ground toward the rise of the sun, and peel or scrape the bark of the roots downward (never upward). After you have enough bark to make a good handful of each, put it in a new earthen crock (the crock dare never have been used), and add two quarts of water and boil down to one pint. After this is done filter and boil the liquid down to a jelly by adding a small quantity of wheat flour so as to form a mass, roll into ordinary sized pills, coating with pulverized sugar or chocolate if desired. Dose, three pills per day. If this remedy does not effect a cure in a very short time, there is no use of resorting to others, as the worst kind of cases have been cured by this remedy.

A VERY GOOD REMEDY FOR WHITE SWELLING.

Add one quart of unslacked lime to two quarts of water, mix well, and let it stand over night. The scum that collect on the lime water must be taken off and a pint of linseed oil added, after which it must be mixed into a consistency of putty. When this is done, add a small quantity of equal parts lard and bees wax, then put it in a pot and boil it well and make plasters. Apply plaster to affected part, renewing every day until swelling is gone. A very good remedy.

COMMENTARY:

White swelling as defined here is the swelling of a joint due to the outburst of fluid in the joint, often a result of tuberculous arthritis.

HOW TO CURE WEAKNESS OF THE LIMBS AND
TO REMOVE GIDDINESS.

Take ten drops of oil of cloves in a tablespoonful of white wine early in the morning before eating anything. This remedy is also applicable to cure the mother pains and colic, or the cold when settled in the bowels, and to stop vomiting. A few drops of this applied to the aching tooth relieves the pain.

A SURE CURE FOR PERSONS WHO CAN'T MAKE THEIR WATER.

Take a red flannel cloth, and after doubling it, urinate on it and apply to the abdomen of the patient as warm as you possibly can. Repeat this as often as it gets cold, and in fifteen or twenty minutes the patient will make his or her water. Bear in mind, this must be done by a male for a female, and by a female for a male. We are pleased to say that this remedy has cured hundreds.

COMMENTARY:

This charm employs an obvious sympathetic component: using the urine of the healer to encourage the patient's body to produce urine by bringing the body in contact with the wetness of it to encourage flow.

A VERY GOOD REMEDY FOR THOSE WHO CAN'T KEEP THEIR WATER.

Take a hog bladder and burn it to a powder. Dose, take a small quantity of the powder internally several times a day.

COMMENTARY:

In like manner to the previous charm, we see sympathetic magic as work through the use of the hog bladder, which is large, to encourage the patient's bladder to be able to retain and hold their water accordingly.

HOW TO PREVENT SWELLING.

Apply a cloth to the swollen parts five or six fold in thickness, dipped in cold water, and when it grows warm renew the wetting. This must be repeated as often as may be deemed necessary, taking into consideration the condition of the patient. An old Indian remedy.

A CURE FOR CANCER IN ITS FIRST STAGES.

Take alum, vinegar, and honey equal quantities, together with wheat flour and make a plaster by mixing the ingredients well together. Apply plaster to the diseased parts, renewing every twenty-four hours.

COMMENTARY:

Please note that no proof shows that any of these ingredients have any effect on any cancer.

A NEVER-FAILING REMEDY FOR MEMBRANEOUS CROUP.

If a child has got the membraneous croup, take one tablespoonful of warm wine and give it to the child inwardly. This will cause the child to throw up the slime and membrane, after which the child will be relieved in a short time. If one dose will not relieve it, give a second dose. If the second dose will not relieve it, give it the third. In many instances one dose is sufficient while on the other hand it takes two or three. This remedy was obtained from an old Indian Doctor.

ANOTHER GOOD REMEDY FOR MEMBRANEOUS CROUP.

Take one teaspoonful of pole-cat's lard, and after melting it, give it to the child inwardly as warm as it can be taken. This will cause the child to vomit, but we guarantee if this remedy does not effect a cure there is no other remedy in existence that will help the child.

ANOTHER FIRST-CLASS REMEDY FOR CROUP, TO BE USED FOR CHILDREN AND ADULTS.

Take one tablespoonful of sugar, one tablespoonful of molasses, one tablespoonful of vinegar and one table-spoonful of pulverized alum. Melt these articles well together and give the patient from one teaspoonful to one tablespoonful as often as may be deemed necessary until a cure is effected.

A GOOD REMEDY FOR VOMITING AND DIARRHEA.

Take pulverized cloves and eat them, together with bread soaked in red wine, and you will soon find relief. The cloves may be put upon the bread.

HOW TO CURE THE CRAMP COLIC IN PERSONS.

Take a white dog tird and pulverize it to a powder; then take one teacupful of sweet milk and add the pulverized dog tird to the sweet milk. After this is done take a charge of gunpowder and add it to the above ingredients, mix well together and let the patient drink it at one time if it can be done.

This remedy has effected a cure in every instance, and where the best physicians could do no more than little children. It can be flavored with vanilla, or anything desired. If one dose does not effect a cure, give the patient the second or third, but this is seldom necessary.

A NEVER-FAILING REMEDY FOR COSTIVENESS.

Take the inner bark of butternut (commonly called white walnut), and scrape or peal the bark off downward (never upward). After this is done take a good handful of the bark and put it in a new earthen crock that has never been used; and one quart of water and boil down to one pint, after which filter and boil liquid down to a jelly by adding wheat flour so as to form a mass. Roll into ordinary size pills, coating with pulverized sugar or chocolate if desired. Dose, three pills for an adult every three hours until operation takes place. Three pills are generally sufficient. If this don't move the bowels there is nothing in existence that will, as it is something similar to quicksilver.

<hr>

HOW TO MAKE A VERY VALUABLE PILL FOR THE LIVER.

Take four ounces of dandelion root, one ounce of mandrake root, two ounces of elecampane root, ten grains of capsicum pepper, and one-half ounce of Prussian aloes. Put these articles in a vessel and add two quarts of water and boil it down to one quart, after which filter and boil liquid down to a jelly by adding wheat flour so as to form a mass. Roll into ordinary sized pill, coating with anything desired. Dose, three pills per day. This remedy will work on the liver and will cure any disease of the same, if followed according to our directions.

<hr>

A GOOD CURE FOR SCABBY HEADS OF CHILDREN.

Take one pound of pickled pork and one pound of cabbage. Boil these articles precisely the same as you would for eating; then skim the substance off and anoint the diseased part of the head with the liquid. This is a sure cure for scabby heads on children, and will heal them if rightly attended.

A CERTAIN CURE FOR BURNS OR SCALDS ON PERSONS OR ANIMALS.

Take sweet oil and mix it with a small quantity of equal parts of pulverized red chalk and white lead; then take a feather and anoint the affected part. This will relieve the pain and heal the sore in a very short time.

A SURE AND NEVER-FAILING CURE FOR SMALL-POX.

The following is a sure and never-failing cure for the small-pox: One ounce of cream of tartar dissolved in a pint of boiling water, to be drunk when cold, at intervals. It can be taken at any time, as a preventative as well as a curative. It is known to have cured thousands of cases without a single failure. Gypsy remedy.

A CERTAIN CURE FOR SUPPRESSED MENSES IN FEMALES.

Take one-half ounce Prussian aloes tinctured, one-half ounce gum marrh, and put it in a three-ounce bottle. After this is done add two ounces of water so that it dissolves. Dose, one teaspoonful three times per day, before meals. Keep on using for three or four weeks, refilling bottle when it gets empty. At the same time take a double handful of verivine roots and put them in a quart of water, and boil down to one pint. A half-cup of tea must be taken with the above preparation. Keep on using these remedies for three or four weeks, and we guarantee it will effect a cure, notwithstanding the fact that the medicine is a little unpleasant to the taste, and that the patient had been treated by the best physicians without getting but very little if any relief. Those who use this remedy will not only feel a thousand times obliged to us for making it known, but will also not regret having invested the trifle for it, as well as the many other equally valuable ones.

ANOTHER GOOD REMEDY FOR SUPPRESSIVE MENSES AND FEMALE WEAKNESS.

Add a good handfull of sarsaparilla root (the root must be cut into small pieces) to one quart of good wine.

Dose, one tablespoonful three times a day, until relief is obtained. A cure is generally in less than a week's time.

A MARVELOUS DISCOVERY REVEALED.

A sure cure for leucorrhea or whites and female weakness.

Take one double handful of little green shad leaves, and after adding two quarts of boiling water, boil down to one pint. Drink a half tea cup of this decoction three times a day for four or five weeks in succession, making a fresh tea every other day. We have refused large sums for this valuable secret time and again, because we have just lately discovered it, and furthermore, so far as our observation goes, it is entirely unknown to the medical profession, therefore, we had no trouble to make more by the sale of the preparation than to sell the secret.

We guarantee this remedy to permanently cure the worst cases of leucorrhoea or whites and female weakness in a very short time. Should the case be chronic we can't guarantee to effect a permanent cure in every instance, but we do guarantee to give more relief in a short time than any other remedy ever heard of. We have permanently cured a number of ladies, so that they have heaven on earth rather than the reverse. Those who are inclined to doubt our word had better write, or come to see us personally, and be convinced that every word we say is true.

So much confidence have we in this remedy that we don't hesitate to treat any one (excepting chronic cases) who sustain the reputation of being honest, and not charge one cent until the patient feels satisfied that she is permanently cured.

Let good doctors and quacks talk about our assertions and book as much as they please. To those we can prove that we have permanently cured cases where some of the best physicians failed to effect a cure.

We make a specialty of treating only a few kinds of disease, and these diseases are the worst flesh and blood can fall heir to. One fact we wish to impress upon the mind of our many readers, and that is, that we never undertake a case unless we are positive of either effecting a permanent cure, or giving relief. Our motto is not to run the risk of killing, or ruining any one for life, nor is it to take any one's hard-erned dollars unless we are deserving of them.

We have still another point we wish to call our readers' attention to, and that is that we cure and have permanently cured the worst kind of cases of gonorrhea. We are not anxious to take cases of this kind unless it is of the worst kind blood and flesh can fall heir to, and such parties we will guarantee a permanent cure (unless entirely too far gone), eradicating everything from the system, so that when one becomes sick later on, it will never return again.

We have not only cured many cases of this kind but have actually saved several from the grave. Anyone desiring further information in regard to this subject, or that of leucorrhea, or whites, and female weakness, and will call on us, or will write us, we will be glad to give further explanation. You will note that we can treat patients as successfully a thousand miles away as if under treatment personally, and that we conduct our own correspondence, which is strictly confidential.

———◆———

A SURE CURE FOR CONSUMPTION, COUGHS AND COLDS.

Take two ounces of sarsaparilla root, two ounces of elecampane root one ounce of horehoud tea, two ounces of hops, two ounces of liverwort root, one ounce of lungwort, one ounce of skunk cabbage, one ounce of little snakeroot, one half of Indian turnip, and one ounce of licorice root. Put all these articles in a cooking kettle, and after adding one gallon of water, boil down to three quarts and filter through a thin cloth, then add two pounds of brown sugar and one ounce of gum arabic, after this is done boil down to a syrup and add one ounce of sulphuric ether or golden tincture. Keep in a tight place, and always shake before using. Dose, a tablespoonful three times a day before meals.

This we don't hesitate to say is the greatest remedy for consumption, cough, and colds before the public today, and it is with the hope that we will not only be the means of many being permanently cured from this dreadful disease, but also that many will be saved from the grave by us making it known. We don't pretend to say that it will entirely cure cases that are chronic, or of too long standing, but we do pretend to say that we don't believe a better remedy to give relief and to prolong the life of those who are afflicted with the disease of long standing can be found.

We can't speak half enough in its favor through our valuable book, but to those who are afflicted with the dreadful disease, either in its first or last stage, we advise to use it, and be convinced that every word we say is true.

A NEVER-FAILING REMEDY FOR MALARIAL FEVER, AGUE, &C.

Take about one half ounce of lobelia (it grows on almost any ridge), and after adding a little water boil down to a strong decoction of tea. Drink the tea in one dose, and if this does not affect a cure, take the second or third, but this is seldom necessary. A teaspoonful of tincture of lobelia may be used, if the tea cannot be obtained. This remedy we guarant our readers will affect a permanent cure in two or three days' time.

A WELL-TRIED REMEDY FOR MINER'S ASTHMA, GIDDINESS IN THE HEAD, COUGHS AND COLD.

Take one quart of good old rye whiskey, three good fresh lemons, and after peeling off both yellow and white skin, cut into small pieces. Beat three eggs well and add to whiskey, together with the lemon and one pound of brown sugar. Mix these articles well together, and also keep the vessels well closed, and always shake before using. Dose, three or four tablespoonfuls each day until permanently cured. This remedy has cured the worst kind of miner's ashma within two months. Those who try it will agree with us when we say that a relief will be felt within a few days, and that this recipe alone is worth more than the cost of the entire book.

A SURE CURE FOR SHORTNESS OF BREATH, GIDDINESS, CROUP, WHOOPING COUGHS AND COLDS, &C.

Take equal parts of honey-suckle blossoms and soft white sugar and put in a good glass jar, or some other vessel that can be closed tight. Mix these articles well together, and after making jar or vessel as tight as possible, stand away in a cool place for three or four weeks, then filter and squeeze substance out of blossoms and add a wine glass full of good brandy to each pint of syrup. Dose for children under two years of age, one-half teaspoonful. Children over two years, one teaspoonful. Adults and half grown persons, one tablespoonful. This may be used as often as may be deemed necessary. For croup take every half hour until relief is obtained. A better remedy than this for the above ailments is not to be found. We do not hesitate to say that fortunes could be made by the sale of this preparation.

A SURE CURE FOR RUPTURE ON CHILDREN OR BEASTS.

Take one double handful of little thorn stem leaves, one double handful of house *marsh*, one double handful of comphery root, one-half pound of sheep tallow or hog's lard and two ounces of rabbit lard. Fry the herbs and roots in the lard or tallow, then filter through a cloth. Anoint affected parts several times a day, each time rubbing in well. Continue on using in this manner for some time, and we feel confident relief will be derived from its use in a short time, and finally a cure. It will also cure rupture on grown persons, if not of too long standing.

HOW TO MAKE A PLASTER TO REMOVE MORTIFICATION ON PERSONS OR ANIMALS.

Take six hen eggs and boil them in hot ashes until they are right hard, then take the yellow of the eggs and fry them in a gill of lard until they are quite black. After this is done add a handful of *rue*, then filter and add a gill of sweet oil. It will take most effect when prepared by a male for a female, and by a female for a male. Bear this in mind.

A GOOD REMEDY FOR REMOVING RHEUMATISM OUT OF JOINTS.

Take oil of linseed, oil of cedar and oil of amber, each one ounce; gum camphor, one-half ounce; dissolved in one-half ounce of sweet oil by rubbing in a mortar, first adding to the camphor a few drops of alcohol, so as to powder it; spirits of turpentine and laundanum, each one ounce; mix and shake well before using. Anoint diseased parts with this lotion as often as desired, each time rubbing in well. Our powwowing method is far superior to this, as it originates from the Scripture, and therefore, we must believe that our Savior's medicine can do more than others.

Our object in suggesting this remedy is simply because it is often a difficult matter to get one to powwow for rhumatism on account of the fact that that party is liable to get the disease, if the constitution is not stronger than the patient's.

HOW TO MAKE A GOOD PLASTER FOR DRAWING BOILS TOGETHER.

Take one handful of sour rumple and wrap it up in green leaves; then put it in hot ashes and roast until it gets soft. After this is done put it on a clean cloth and apply to boils as warm as can be borne. This will draw the boil together and at the same time take the inflammation out, and relieve the pain in a very short time.

A NEVER-FAILING REMEDY FOR REMOVING WARTS.

Take as many little stones as you have warts and rub them well with the stones, then take them to some cemetery and cast them in a grave before the corpse is buried. Do this in the decrease of the moon and you can rest assured that your warts will soon disappear. This we consider a valuable secret to those who have warts on their person.

ANOTHER MARVELOUS DISCOVERY! A WELL-TRIED REMEDY FOR RUNNING ULCERS AND WOUNDS OF LONG STANDING.

Take carpenter's glue and boil it down to a thick paste, then make a good plaster and apply to ulcer or wound of long standing, and we guarantee this will draw the corruption or foul matter from the ulcer or wound of long standing and heal it up in a very short time.

Bear in mind that a small hole must be cut in the plaster so as to emit the corruption or foul matter from the running wound. Add a new plaster as often as may be deemed necessary.

We consider this information worth ONE HUNDRED DOLLARS to any physician or person afflicted with this terrible disease. Those who desire additional information in regard to this subject will write us, sending stamp for a reply, we will take pleasure to give further explanation.

Mr. Steel has cured a running ulcer on his leg that was contracted in the Army thirty years ago, and which five of the best physicians of this vicinity failed to cure after trying a great many remedies.

A SURE CURE FOR TUMORS ON CATTLE.

Take any bone which you accidentally find (you dare not be looking for it) and rub the tumor with it, always bearing in mind that this must be done in the decrease of the moon, and the tumor will certainly disappear. The bone, however, must be replaced as it was found.

A CERTAIN CURE FOR HOLLOW HORNS ON COWS.

Bore a small hole in the horn of the cow, and inject a small quantity of her last milk. After this is done tar the horn or horns well and tie shut.

A VERY GOOD REMEDY FOR RING BONES ON HORSES.

Put unslacked lime in a bag and tie it around the ring bone as tight as you possibly can, then keep pouring warm water on the lime for a short time. The horse will get uneasy when the lime begins to slack, but keep it on as long as you can, as this will kill the ring bone on the horse.

A SURE CURE FOR SWENEY IN HORSES.

Rub the diseased part with a toad until it dies. This must be done on the first Friday in the decrease of the moon for the first time. Repeat this again on the second Friday of the decrease of the moon, and also on the first Friday of the increase of the moon. This remedy permanently cures, after all others fail. A Gypsy cure.

ANOTHER REMEDY FOR SWENEY IN HORSES.

Take one ounce of oil of spike, one ounce of oil of stone, and one ounce of oil of juniper. Mix all these ingredients together, then take a feather and anoint the diseased part as often as may be deemed necessary until a cure is effected.

A FIRST-CLASS REMEDY FOR WIND COLIC IN HORSES.

Take your left shoe and urinate in it, then pour the urine out of the shoe into the right ear of the horse. After this is done urinate in the right shoe and pour the urine out of the right shoe into the left ear of the horse. This will cause the horse to shake itself more or less, but we guarantee the wind colic will leave the horse, and also that a cure will be the result.

———❖———

A WELL-TRIED REMEDY FOR
BOUND-UP HORSES.

Take a quantity of the inner bark of butternut (commonly call white walnut), and after adding one gallon of water to it, boil down to two quarts of strong solution. Dose, pour one pint into the horse, and if the bowels do not move within half an hour, repeat the second time; if the second dose will not work on the horse, repeat the third time, if the third does not take effect, give the fourth, and if the fourth will not move the bowels of the horse, there is no other remedy in existence that will, as this remedy is something similar to quicksilver. In many instances it is not necessary to give the horse more than the first or second dose, while on the other hand it takes three and four. The fourth dose either effects a cure or kills.

———❖———

HOW TO CURE HEAVINESS IN HORSES.

Take a quantity of *skunk* cabbage root (commonly called pole cat cabbage), equal part mullen leaves and one-fourth pound of ground ginger. Boil these articles well, and give one-half pint with their feed three times a day for two or three weeks. This we assure our readers will cure the worst cases of heaviness. Bear in mind the horse dare not be fed dusty hay, or overheated while under this treatment.

ANOTHER REMEDY FOR BOUND-UP HORSES.

Take a small quantity of warm water and soap, and make a strong solution of soap suds. Inject soap suds into the horse and this will cause the bowels to move. We never heard of, or found this remedy to fail, if resorted to in time.

A VERY GOOD REMEDY TO DRY UP WOUNDS ON HORSES OR PERSONS.

Take old leather (of old boots or shoes is preferable), and burn them to a coal; then pulverize to a powder and sprinkle it on the sore or wound. This we assure our readers will dry up any wound in a short time. The wound or sore should be washed occasionally with castile soap, and rinsed with cold water. This remedy has been used successfully in the army by one of the authors, who never knew or heard of it failing.

COMMENTARY:

With this charm, the sympathetic measure taken is with leather standing in as the skin of the wound, which is dried and burnt to a crisp to likewise dry out the wound and rid the body of any wet-natured infection. This was probably used by Issac D. Steel during his time in the Civil War, likely during his enlistment in Company G for the Pennsylvania 7th Calvary in winter 1864, where he served as a private for over a year.

HOW TO MAKE A FIRST-CLASS HORSE POWDER.

Take one-half pound of foenugreek powder, one-half pound of sulphur, one-half pound cream of tartar, one-half pound saltpeter, one-half pound of powdered sassafras bark, two ounces of gun poweder, two ounces of pulverized kimell seed, four ounces of burnt leather, powdered, two ounces of hickory wood ashes, two ounces of wheat bran, two ounces of sour dough and one-half pound of powdered antimony.

Mix these articles well together and we don't hesitate to say that a better powder you never had in your life. Dose, one tablespoonful mixed in their feed three times a week is sufficient. Should the animal be sick, add a tablespoonful each day for a short time, always bearing in mind that the feed must be made wet before adding the powder.

Five dollars has often been refused for this recipe.

It was obtained from an old horse doctor who practiced in the United States army thirty years ago. It is not necessary for us to say that when this powder is once introduced there will be but very little room in the market for other powders.

A REMARKABLE REMEDY.

I. D. Steel's Army Liniment [3]

This valuable remedy was discovered by I. D. Steel while in the army during the late war, having been obtained by him from some of the most renowned medical men in the world, who used it a great deal in their practice.

The Army Liniment is one of the most powerful remedies ever known or prepared for man or beast, curing the worst cases of rheumatism, pains in the back, sprains, swellings, bruises, and cuts—will keep cold out of cuts and wounds, and heal all descriptions of sores and wounds on men or beasts—cures headache, earache, toothache, sore or swelled throat, and all similar diseases.

The Army Liniment is also highly recommended for fresh wounds, stiffness, sprains, bruises, stiff joints and all similar diseases in horses, mules, and other stock.

---

3   I. D. Steel is identified as one of the authors, Issac D. Steel.

RECIPE FOR MAKING I.D. STEEL'S ARMY LINIMENT.

To make one gallon Liniment, take one ounce of castile soap and put it in a vessel and add one or two gills of warm water and shake it, until it is dissolved to a liniment, then put four ounces of beef gall in it and two ounces of dog lard or goose oil, one ounce coal oil, two ounces balsam de maltha, one ounce of tincture balsam of rue or cowry, two ounces opedeldoc, two ounces British oil, two ounces spirits of turpentine, four ounces opium or laudanum, four ounes aqua ammonia, four ounces tincture of camphor, some tincture of aloes to give color, and one half pint of alcohol, then shake it well until it is dissolved. Let is stand a day or so, then divide it equally and put in four quart bottles filling them with warm water. If not sufficiently colored, add more tincture of aloes, then let is stand a few days and cork afterwards. Shake well before using.

Directions

For Rheumatism—Bathe the parts affected and rub well, drying it in at the fire or warm stove. For pains in back or sprains, apply in same manner as for rheumatism. For toothache, rub the cheek and temple well with the liniment and put some in the tooth. For earache, drop a few drops in the ear. For headache, rub the forehead and temples well for from fifteen to twenty minutes. For sore or swelled throat, apply to the throat. For fresh wounds and cuts, bruises, sprains, stiff joints, &c., in man or beasts, apply the liniment to the parts affected three times a day, rubbing in well. Continue to bathe the affected parts until relief is obtained.

HOW TO MAKE A FIRST-CLASS LINIMENT FOR SWENEY, SPRAINS, BRUISES, STIFF JOINTS AND ALL KINDS OF CUTS AND BROKEN BONES, &C., TO BE USED FOR PERSONS OR ANIMALS.

Take one pound of old smoked bacon (the older the better) and one handful of comphery root; cut these articles fine and put them in a frying pan together with one quart of water; boil substance out of bacon and root, then filter and add ten cents' worth each of oil of stone and oil of spike. Bottle and keep well corked. Apply to the afflicted parts as often as desired, always bearing in mind that the patient should get as close to the heat as can be borne, so that the liniment will soak in the skin more readilty. We have cured horses that had stiff joints in the legs of six and eight years standing.

HOW TO MAKE A VERY GOOD HEALING SALVE.

Take one double handfull of balsam buds, four ounes of sheep tallow, two ounces of beeswax and two ounces of pitch pine sap. Fry substance out of these articles, then filter through a clean cloth. A better salve for healing wounds of every description we don't believe can be found.

ANOTHER GOOD REMEDY FOR THE BITE OF SNAKE.

Take one pint of the substance of strong bacon, one tea-spoonful of salt. The white of four eggs well beaten and after mixing these articles well together apply to the wound within twenty-four hours. This will effect a cure.

HOW TO MAKE INDIAN PAIN KILLER.

Take one quart of alcohol, two ounces of spirits of turpentine, two ounces of aqua ammonia, three ounces of gum camphor, one ounce of castile soap, cut fine; two ounces of red capsicum pepper. Mix these articles in a vessel and let stand twelve hours. Shaking it occasionally. Then filter it through a cloth until clear. After this is done add two ounces of oil of sassafras and one-half ounce of oil of winter-green. Dose for an adult fifteen to thirty drops according to constitution and condition of patient. Give children in proportion to age.

This remedy is intended to relieve pain externally or internally.

HOW TO MAKE FIRST-CLASS CHOLERA MORBUS AND DIARRHOEA DROPS.

Take one-half pint adulterated alcohol, one ounce tincture of camphor, one-half ounce of laudanum and one ounce tincture of red capsicum pepper. Mix well together and add a little red color for coloring. Dose for an adult, twenty to thirty drops, in water, every half-hour if deemed necessary. Give children in proprtion to age.

HOW TO MAKE CHOLERA MORBUS AND DIARRHOEA PILLS.

Take one ounce of gum camphor, ten grains of opium, and mix in a mortar, then roll into ordinary size pills, coating with pulverized sugar or chocolate if desired. Dose, three pills per day. This remedy has been used in the army with great success.

———————

HOW TO MAKE A GOOD LINIMENT FOR NEURALGIA.

Take castile soap one ounce, chloroform one drachm, tincture of aconite one drachm, and one ounce of sulphuric ether. Mix well together and apply to the affected parts as often as desired.

———————

HOW TO MAKE UNITED STATES ARMY NEURALGIA PILLS.

Take three grains strychnine, small quantity of pulverized licorice, and enough gum arabic so as to form a mortar. Roll in twenty-one ordinary sized pills. The pills may be coated with pulverized sugar or anything else desired. Dose, one pill three times a day. Bear in mind these pills are for adults only. The first dose will make the patient feel a little dizzy, but we guarantee if this remedy will not permanently cure neuralgia, there is no other remedy that will work.

HOW TO MAKE A GOOD PLASTER FOR DRAWING PAIN OUT OF THE BODY.

Take the inner bark of butternut (commonly called white walnut) and pound it fine; then take a little sour dough and a little cider vinegar, and after mixing these articles well together make a good plaster.

Take a red flannel rag and wash the afflicted part with vinegar before applying the plaster. This plaster is far superior to that bought in the drug stores, as it draws pain in less than ten or fifteen minutes.

A CERTAIN CURE FOR YELLOW JAUNDICE.

Take a large carrot and hollow it out, then let the person afflicted with the disease urinate in it, and set it away. This will cause the yellow jaundice to disappear as the urine absorbs.

HOW TO MAKE MOTHER DROPS.

Take three ounces of alcohol, thirty drops of laudanum, one half ounce of sulphuric ether, thirty drops of tincture of hops and thirty drops of asafoetida. Mix well together and add a little red color for coloring. Shake well before using. Dose, twenty to thirty drops, according to constitution of patient.

———⋄⋆⋄———

HOW TO MAKE A VERY GOOD PILL FOR SICK HEADACHE AND NEURALGIA.

Take a small quantity of pulverized mandrake root or extracts of mandrake root, together with equal parts powdered aloes, red capsicum pepper, wheat flour and burnt poke root. Mix these articles well together, and add a little gum arabic so as to form a mass, then roll in ordinary size pills, coating with pulverized sugar or anything that may be deemed necessary. Dose, three pills a day. This remedy never failed in curing the worst cases of sick headache.

COMMENTARY:

Neuralgia here is intermittent pain along a nerve, mostly occurring in the head or face but sometimes the neck as well. Likewise, we also see the mention of mandrake root, which is likely referring to one of my favorite plants, the American Mandrake (*Podophyllum peltatum*) or Mayapple, as we call it in Appalachia.

HOW TO MAKE PLASTER FOR BURNS AND SCALDS.

Take one half teacupful of fresh hog's lard, one-half tea-cupful of wheat flour, and mix these articles well together. Spread the salve on a cloth and apply to the affected part, renewing as often as it gets dry. This will cause the fire to draw out and also prevent inflammation from setting in the wound.

ANOTHER METHOD OF CURING BURNS AND SCALDS.

Mix in a bottle ounces of olive oil and four ounces of lime water. Apply this mixture to the affected parts five or six times a day with a feather.

HOW TO GRADUALLY REDUCE THE FLESH.

A strong decoction of sassafras drank frequently will reduce the flesh as reapidly as any remedy known. A strong infusion is made at the rate of an ounce of sassafras to about six gills of water. Boil it slowly for twenty or twenty-five minutes and let it stand to cool, heat it again if desired. Be careful so as not to drink too much.

HOW TO STOP BLEEDING AT THE LUNGS.

Eat freely of raw table salt, or take one teaspoonful three times a day of equal parts of loaf sugar and resin.

HOW TO MAKE A DELICIOUS SUMMER DRINK— THE HEALTHIEST DRINK IN USE.

Put two pounds of white sugar in a crock, pour in a full pint of hot water, add half ounce of baking soda, and mix well together, then beat the white of two eggs well and add half tablespoonful of wheat flour. After mixing these articles well together, add a half teaspoonful of essence of lemon, (or any other flavor desired), one half ounce of tartaric acid, with half a pint of cold water and one gill of cider vinegar. This is sufficient for one hundred and twenty-five glasses of drink.

—————⊷∙⊶—————

A VERY GOOD WAY TO CAUSE CHILDREN TO CUT THEIR TEETH WITHOUT PAIN.

Boil the brain of a rabbit and rub the gums of the children with it and their teeth will grow without pain to them.

COMMENTARY:

An obvious use of sympathy, using the rabbit's brain to rub the gums with hopes that the children's teeth will grow to be as strong as that of a rabbit, whose teeth are naturally superior due to their eating habits and lifestyle.

—————⊷∙⊶—————

A VERY GOOD REMEDY FOR SLEEPLESS PERSONS.

Make a tea of Jerusalem oak and drink it as you would any other tea before going to bed.

—————⊷∙⊶—————

HOW TO CURE CORNS.

Take night shade, bruise and boil it in hog's lard, and anoint the corns with the salve as often as desired until relief is obtained.

———⊷●⊶———

A GOOD CURE FOR PILES.

Take three cigars and a handful of the inner bark of elder, and after rubbing fine add a gill of hog's lard and boil down to an ointment. When it gets cold anoint the affected part as often as may be deemed necessary until a cure is effected.

———⊷●⊶———

A SURE CURE FOR FROST BITTEN.

Take pulverized alum and dissolve in warm water, and apply it to the affected parts until relief is obtained.

———⊷●⊶———

HOW TO CURE PIMPLES AND BLOTCHES.

Take aqua ammonia, tincture of lobelia and tincture of myrrh, each one ounce. Mix well and anoint pimples and blotches four or five times a day until a cure is effected.

HOW TO REMOVE GREASE SPOTS.

Take alcohol, two ounces; urine, two ounces, and aqua ammonia, one ounce; mix and with a bit of woolen cloth wet with this liquid and rub the spot till you get out the grease. This is an excellent preparation for cleaning clothes of grease and other dirt spots.

HOW TO MAKE A REMEDY FOR PURIFYING THE BLOOD, BUILDING UP THE SYSTEM AND TO REMOVE GIDDINESS AND YELLOW COMPLEXION.

Take two ounces of sarsaparilla root, one ounce of blood root, two ounces of dandelion root, one ounce of mandrake root, two ounces of burdock root and one ounce of Virginia snake root. Put these roots in a cooking kettle, and after adding two quarts of water, boil down to one quart of thick solution, then filter through a clean cloth, and boil the liquid a little while longer, after which add either a half pint of good liquor or adulterated alcohol.

Dose, one tablespoonful three times a day. This remedy is equal if not better than all the blood purifying medicines on the market to-day.

HOW TO MAKE A GOOD COUGH SYRUP.

Put one quart of hoarhound to one quart of water, and boil it down to a pint; add two or three sticks of licorice and a tablespoonful of essence of lemon. Dose, take a tablespoonful of the syrup three times a day, or as often as the cough may be troublesome. This is a valuable recipe, and we don't hesitate to say that a great deal of money could be made by the sale of this preparation.

HOW TO MAKE MAGNETIC TOOTHACHE DROPS.

Take equal parts of camphor, sulphuric ether, ammonia, laudanum, tincture of cayenne, and one eight part oil of cloves. Mix well together, saturate with the liquid a small piece of cotton, and apply to the cavity of the diseased tooth, and the pain will cease almost immediately.

HOW TO MAKE A GOOD MEDICINE FOR SORE LUNGS, AND A SURE CURE FOR SPITTING BLOOD.

Take black cohosh, one-half ounce; lobelia, one-quarter ounce; canker root, three-quarters of an ounce; blackberry root, one-third of an ounce; sarsaparilla, one ounce; pleurisy root, one-half of an ounce; steeped in three pints of water. Dose, one tablespoonful three times a day before eating.

RARE AND VALUABLE SECRETS

AND

PRACTICAL RECIPES

HOW TO MAKE A SELF-SHINING STOVE POLISH.

Take plumbago (black lead), finely pulverized, and with a damp woolen rag, dip in the plumbago, and apply to the stove, then polish with a dry cloth, and a most beautiful polish will appear.

HOW TO MAKE A POWDER FOR CLEANING ALL KINDS OF METAL, GLASS, &C.

Take four pounds of best quality whiting (Gilder's is preferable), one-fourth pound good cream tartar and three ounces calcined magnesia; mix thoroughly together, box and label.

Directions

Use the polish dry, with a piece of chamois skin or cotton flannel previously moistened with water or alcohol, and finish with the polish dry. A few moments' rubbing will develop a surprising lustre, different from the polish produced by any other substance.

This is one of the most saleable articles of the day, and something that near every houeskeeper will buy. It is used for gold and silverplated ware, German silver, brass, copper, glass, tin, steel, or any material where a brilliant lustre is required.

It can be put in two ounce paste-board boxes, costs two cents to manufacture, sells readily at retail for fifteen cents. To stores for five or six dollars per hundred boxes. Note the immense profit.

ANOTHER METHOD OF MAKING A FIRST-CLASS POLISH FOR CLEANING ALL KINDS OF METAL, GLASS, &C.

Take ten pound of Gilder's whiting, equal parts of alcohol, aqua ammonia and solution of sal soda. Add these articles to the whiting, together with enough warm water so as to form a mortar. Mix well together, always bearing in mind that the whiting must be finely pulverized, then roll into balls the size of an egg, or as large as desired and put them in an oven to dry.

Each ball costs less than half a cent to manufacture, sells readily at retail for ten cents per ball or three for twenty-five cents. Well worth five dollars to those who desire to travel and make a business of this.

HOW TO MAKE GOLD AND SILVER INK.

Take honey and gold leaf equal parts, triturate until the gold is reduced to the finest possible state of division, agitate with thirty parts hot water, and allow it to settle. Decant the water and repeat the washing several times, finally dry the gold and mix it with a little gum water for use.

Silver Ink—For silver ink the process is the same as gold, substituting the silver leaf for the gold leaf.

HOW TO MAKE A GOOD FURNITURE POLISH.

Take alcohol ninety-eight per cent., one pint, gum copal and shellac, of each one ounce, dragon's blood, one-half ounce. Mix and dissolve by setting in a warm place.

HOW TO MAKE A FIRST-CLASS BAY RUM.

Take oil of bay, fine, one and one-half drachms, oil of ner oli (bigard), ten drops, ether, acetic, two drachms, alcohol, deoderized, three pints, water, two and one-half pints, caromel, sufficient to tinge. Let is stand two weeks and filter.

HOW TO MAKE A MOTH AND FRECKLE LOTION FOR THE SKIN AND COMPLEXION.

Distill two handfuls of jassamine flowers in a quart of rose water and a quart of orange water. Strain through porous paper and add a scruple of musk and a scruple of ambergris. A splendid wash for the skin.

HOW TO MAKE A LOTION FOR CURLING THE HAIR.

Take one pound olive oil, one drachm oil of origanum, one and one-half drachms oil of rosemary. Mix well and apply twice a day. This will curl the straightest hair, if not cut too short.

HOW TO MAKE A HAIR RESTORATIVE AND INVIGORATOR FOR A TRIFLING COST.

Take sugar of lead, borax and lac sulphur, of each one ounce; aqua ammonia one-half ounce; alcohol, one gill. Mix and let stand eighteen hours; then add bay rum, one gill; fine table salt, one tablespoon; soft water, three pints;

essence of bergamot, one ounce. This preparation not only gives a beautiful gloss, but will cause hair to grow upon bald heads arising from all common causes, and turning gray hair to a darker color.

Manner of Application

When the hair is thin or bald, make two applications daily, until this amount is used up; work it into the roots of the hair with a soft brush, or the ends of the fingers, rubbing well each time.

HOW TO MAKE A CEMENT FOR MENDING CHINA, GLASS OR WOODENWARE.

Take one pound of the best white glue, one-half pound dry white lead, one quart soft water, one- half pint alcohol, put the three articles in a dish and that dish in a pot of boiling water let it boil until dissolved, then add the alcohol, and boil again until mixed. A little camphor should be added to preserve it and disguise its composition.

HOW TO CUT AND BORE HOLES IN GLASS.

Any hard steel tool will cut glass with great facility when kept freely wet with camphor dissolved in turpentine. A drill bow may be used, or even the hand alone. A hole bored may readily be enlarged by a round file. The ragged edges of glass vessels may also be thus easily smoothed by a flat file. Flat window glass can be readily sawed by a watch-spring saw by aid of this solution. In short, the most brittle glass can be wrought almost as easily as brass by the use of cutting tools kept constantly moist with camphorized oil of turpentine.

HOW TO MAKE A SILVER PLATING FLUID.

Take an ounce of precipitate of silver to one-half ounce of cyanate of potash and one-fourth ounce of hydro-sulphate of soda; put all in a quart of water, add a little whiting, and shake before using. Apply with a soft rag. A very valuable secret.

HOW TO WRITE SECRET LETTERS.

Put five cents' worth of citrate of potassia in an ounce vial of clear cold water. This forms an invisible fluid. Let it dissolve, and one can use on paper of any color. Use a goose quill in writing. When you wish the writing to become visible, hold it to a red-hot stove.

HOW TO MAKE STICKY FLY PAPER.

Boil linseed oil and resin, melt and add honey; soak the paper in a strong solution of alum, then dry before applying the above.

Agents can make money by selling this article from house to house, as it only cost a trifle to manufacture.

HOW TO MAKE A GOOD BAKING POWDER.

Take one pound tartaric acid in crystals, one and one-half pounds of bi-carbonate of soda, and one and one-half pounds of potato starch; each must be powdered separately. Well dried by a slow heat, well mixed through a sieve. Pack hard in tinfoil, tin, or paper glazed on the outside. With these directions anyone can make as good a baking powder as is sold anywhere. This we consider a valuable secret, and especially to families, as it only costs a trifle to manufacture enough for one year's use.

ANOTHER METHOD OF MAKING A GOOD FURNITURE POLISH.

Take equal parts sweet oil and vinegar, and a pint of gum arabic finely powdered. Shake the bottle and apply the polish with a rag. This will make furniture look almost as good as new.

HOW TO MAKE A FIRST-CLASS LEATHER CEMENT.

Take gutta percha, cut in chloroform to right thickness for use. Equal to Cook's best for putting patches on leather, cloth, shoes or boots.

HOW TO MAKE RED SEALING WAX.

Take four pounds shellac, one and one-half pounds venier turpentine, three pounds finest cinnebar, and add four ounces venetian. Mix the whole well together and melt over a very slow fire. Pour it on a thick, smooth glass, or any other flat, smooth surface, and make it into three or five or ten cent sticks.

HOW TO MAKE COLOGNE.

Take one gallon ninety-five per cent alcohol, or cologne spirits, two ounces oil of bergamot, one-half ounce of orange, one-half ounce of oil of cedar, one drachm oil of nevoi, one-half drachm oil of rosemary. Mix well and it is for for use.

HOW TO MAKE A GOOD WRITING FLUID.

Dissolve a small quantity of aniline, black, (or any other color desired), in as much boiling water as may be deemed necessary. This makes an excellent writing fluid, and costs less than a half cent per bottle to manufacture. Agents can make money by the sale of this preparation, as a gallon of the best writing fluid can be made for less than ten cents.

A CERTAIN CURE FOR DRUNKENNESS.

Take sulphate of iron, five grains; magnesia, ten grains; peppermint water, eleven drachms; spirits of nutmeg, one drachm, three times a day. This preparation acts as a tonic and stimulant, and so partially supplies the place of the accustomed liquor, and prevents that absolute physical and moral prostration that follows a sudden breaking off from the use of stimulating drinks.

THE END.

LIST OF REMEDIES

About the Author

Jake Richards holds his Appalachian-Melungeon heritage close to his blood and bones. His family heritage in Appalachia goes back generations; they have lived in southwest Virginia, east Tennessee, and the western Carolinas for a good four hundred years. He spent most of his childhood at his great-grandmother's house on Big Ridge in North Carolina, wading the waters of the Watauga and traipsing the mountains by his ancestral home on the ridge. "My family," Jake writes, "always spoke of the old wives' tales and folk remedies. They were mountain people to the bone; hunters, farmers, faith healers, preachers, and root-diggers." Jake has practiced Appalachian folk magic for over a decade. Aside from being an author and practitioner, Jake is a member of the Melungeon Heritage Association, holds a seat on the board of WAM: We Are Melungeons, and is the creator of HOM: House of Malungia, Melungeon cultural society. You can find him on Instagram *@jake_richards13*